Modern Practical Nursing Series

This important nursing series, designed specifically for the
State Enrolled Nurse and Pupil Nurse is published as a 'parent'
book covering the basic skills entitled AN OUTLINE OF BASIC
NURSING CARE, and a number of smaller handbooks covering
the individual specialities as the nurse is moved from one
discipline to another.

The following volumes are available;

Parent Book: AN OUTLINE OF BASIC NURSING CARE

Elizabeth M. Welsh, R.G.N., R.N.T.
*Director of Nursing and Midwifery Education, Northern Ireland
Council for Nurses and Midwives.*
Mary Gillespie, R.F.N., R.G.N., R.C.I.,
*Clinical Instructor, Teaching Division, Glasgow Royal Infirmary,
and Associated Hospitals.*
Catherine Asher, R.G.N., S.C.M., R.N.T.
*Senior Nursing Officer, Teaching Division, Glasgow Royal
Infirmary and Associated Hospitals.*

224 pages   220 illustrations   £1.00 net

Volume 1: PAEDIATRIC ORTHOPAEDICS

Mary I. Gilchrist, R.S.C.N., R.G.N., O.N.C.
*Ward Sister, Royal Hospital for Sick Children, Drumchapel Branch,
Glasgow.*
Noel J. Blockey, F.R.C.S., M.(
Consultant Orthopaedic Surge
Drumchapel Branch, Glasgow.

112 pages   2(

GW00691608

Volume 2: THEATRE ROU

Morag H. Campbell, R.G.N.,
Senior Nursing Officer (Thec
Infirmary.

160 pages   (

Volume 3: PAEDIATRIC SURGERY

Elizabeth D. Strathdee, S.R.N., R.S.C.N.
Ward Sister, Royal Hospital for Sick Children, Glasgow.
D.G. Young, M.B., Ch.B., F.R.C.S. (Edin), D.T.M. & H.
Senior Lecturer in Paediatric Surgery, The University, Glasgow.
*Honorary Consultant Surgeon, Royal Hospital for Sick Children,
Glasgow.*

96 pages   30 illustrations   £0.60 net

Volume 4: DERMATOLOGY

A. Keenan, R.G.N., S.C.M.
Ward Sister, Glasgow Royal Infirmary.
J. O'D. Alexander, M.B., Ch.B., F.R.C.P.
Consultant Dermatologist, Glasgow Royal Infirmary.

96 pages   34 black & white,   £0.75 net
                          24 colour illustrations

Volume 5: UROLOGY.

Margaret W. A. Stirling, R.G.N., S.C.M.
Ward Sister, Urological Department, Glasgow Royal Infirmary.
Roy Scott, M.B., Ch.B., F.R.C.S. (Glas.), F.R.C.S. (Ed.).
Consultant Urologist, Glasgow Royal Infirmary.

80 pages   17 illustrations   £0.65 net

Volume 6: PLASTIC SURGERY AND BURNS TREATMENT

Ian T. Jackson, M.B., Ch.B., F.R.C.S. (Glas.), F.R.C.S. (Ed.).
*Consultant Plastic Surgeon, Glasgow & West of Scotland Regional
Plastic and Oral Surgery Service, Canniesburn Hospital, Bearsden,
Glasgow.*
E.S. Macallan, R.G.N., S.C.M., Plastic Surgery Cert.
*Former Ward Sister, Glasgow and West of Scotland Regional Plastic
and Oral Surgery Service, Canniesburn Hospital, Bearsden, Glasgow.
At present a member of the Teaching Staff in the School of Nursing,
Glasgow Royal Infirmary and Associated Hospitals.*

160 pages   90 illustrations   £0.60 net

Volume 7: PSYCHIATRY.

Emily A. Lee, R.G.N., R.M.N., R.C.I. (Edin.).
*Glasgow Royal Infirmary and Associated Hospitals Teaching
Department, Clinical Instructor based at Eastern District Hospital,
Glasgow.*
A.B. Sclare, M.B., Ch.B., F.R.C.P. (Glas.), F.R.C.P. (Edin.),
M.R.C.P. (Lond.), D.P.M.
*Consultant Psychiatrist, Eastern District Hospital and Glasgow
Royal Infirmary. Mackintosh Lecturer in Psychological Medicine,
University of Glasgow.*

192 pages   £0.60 net

Volume 8: ORTHOPAEDIC SURGERY

Thomas H. Norton, M.B., Ch.B., F.R.C.S.E.
*Consultant Orthopaedic Surgeon to Victoria Infirmary and
Philipshill Orthopaedic Hospital, Glasgow.*
Judith M. Tait, S.C.M., O.N.C., R.N.T.
*Senior Nursing Officer, Teaching Division, Glasgow Royal Infirmary
School of Nursing.*

148 pages   128 two-colour illustrations   £0.90 net

Volume 9: ADULT MEDICINE

E.H.R. Laird, R.G.N., S.C.M., H.V. Cert.
Unit Nursing Officer, Glasgow Royal Infirmary.
R.D. Barr, M.B., Ch.B., M.R.C.P.
Registrar, Medical Department, Glasgow Royal Infirmary.

144 pages   21 illustrations   £0.65 net

11 | Modern
Practical
Nursing
Series

Medical Paediatrics

William B. Doig, M.B., Ch.B., M.R.C.P.
(Edinburgh and Glasgow), D.C.H.
Consultant Paediatric Cardiologist, Royal Hospital for Sick Children, Glasgow.

Alison Montford, R.S.C.N., R.G.N.
Formerly Ward Sister, Royal Hospital for Sick Children, Glasgow.

WILLIAM HEINEMANN MEDICAL BOOKS LIMITED:
LONDON

This book is dedicated to Andrew and
Justine

First Published 1972
© Alison Montford and W. B. Doig 1972
ISBN 0 433 07694 1
Printed in Great Britain by
Redwood Press Limited
Trowbridge, Wiltshire

Contents

		History of Medical Paediatrics	1
Chapter	*1*	Where Do our Patients Come from	3
Chapter	*2*	General Aspects of a Medical Ward	7
Chapter	*3*	A Few Points about the Normal Child	8
Chapter	*4*	Infant Feeding	12
Chapter	*5*	Common Investigations	16
Chapter	*6*	Investigations Involving Simple Observation	18
Chapter	*7*	Investigations Involving Urinalysis	19
Chapter	*8*	Investigations Involving Blood Examination	23
Chapter	*9*	Lumbar Puncture	27
Chapter 10		X-ray Examinations	29
Chapter 11		Medical Diseases of Children	31
Chapter 12		Alimentary Diseases	32
Chapter 13		Mechanical Faults	35
Chapter 14		Faults in Digestion	38
Chapter 15		Some Infections of the Alimentary Tract	42
Chapter 16		Failure to Thrive in Infants	45
Chapter 17		Vitamin Deficiency Diseases	49
Chapter 18		Diseases Affecting the Urinary Tract	51
Chapter 19		Some Common Diseases of the Renal Tract	52
Chapter 20		Disorders of the Cardiovascular System	56
Chapter 21		Blood Disorders	65

Chapter 22	Malignant Diseases of Children	71
Chapter 23	Diseases of the Respiratory System	75
Chapter 24	Infections of the Lower Respiratory Tract	81
Chapter 25	Disorders of the Nervous System	87
Chapter 26	Convulsions	92
Chapter 27	Meningitis	94
Chapter 28	Cerebral Palsy	96
Chapter 29	Diabetes Mellitus	98
Chapter 30	Jaundice	100
	Paediatric Line-Up	
Chapter 31	Words to the Nurse	104
Chapter 32	The Paediatric Nurse	105
Chapter 33 1	Reporting	108
Chapter 34	The Dying Child	109
Chapter 35	General Care of Children—Hygiene	110
Chapter 36	General Care of Children—Feeding	113
Chapter 37	Administration of Oral Medicines	120
Chapter 38	Giving Injections	123
Chapter 39	T.P.R.	124
Chapter 40	Prevention of Accidents	128
Chapter 41	Weighing and Measuring Children	130
Chapter 42	Collection of Urine Specimens	132
Chapter 43	Collection of Stools	136
Chapter 44	Serving Meals	138
Chapter 45	Special Diets	143
Chapter 46	Intravenous Fluids	146
Chapter 47	Oxygen Therapy	148
Chapter 48	Infectious Diseases	151
Chapter 49	Dismissal from Hospital	153
	Acknowledgements	154
	Index	155

Foreword

This book has been written by a ward sister, and a physician in one of the most famous hospitals for sick children in the world.

Following a short history tracing the growth of medical paediatrics there is a section planned to help the nurse understand what is wrong with her small patient.

A two-page insert shows the team working together to make illness, convalescence and cure smooth and effective.

A nursing section follows to complete an all-round practical book for nurses in training in Medical Paediatric wards.

No ward is perfect—but there is a great deal in every ward the student nurse must remember. Some blank pages have been left in this book so that you can jot down any particularly good ideas which you wish to remember.

A. M.
W. D.

There are two other books in this series devoted to paediatrics:-

MPNS 1: PAEDIATRIC ORTHOPAEDICS by Mary I. Gilchrist and Noel J. Blockey and

MPNS 3: PAEDIATRIC SURGERY by Elizabeth D. Strathdee and Daniel G. Young.

History of Medical Paediatrics

Paediatrics is a well established branch of medicine nowadays. The sick child is readily accommodated in hospitals or units designed specifically to care for his needs and staffed by people who are particularly interested in his health and welfare. But it was not always so.

It is just over a century ago that hospitals began to pay any real concern to the child's particular needs by opening wards for him in general hospitals. Prior to this children who were not born into financially secure homes led a sorry life. Many died in infancy: those who survived to an age when today's child might be starting school would more than likely be exploited by miserable hard labour in poorly paid employment in Dickensian conditions. If ill-health overtook them not only would they lose their employment and thus be no longer an asset to their family, but no one would care for their physical and mental needs.

About the time of the Industrial Revolution the lot of the British child was probably at its most dismal: no education, no welfare and no medical care. Fortunately social revolution began to better the child's lot. Managers of factories and mines in addition to using child labour also gradually learnt to care for them. Schools were set up in the factories. Physical illness was recognised and clinics and dispensaries began to open. The sick child was no longer doomed to beg, and cope with destitution.

By the beginning of this century the Universities had begun to teach and instruct on the medical care of children and so more hospitals and children's wards came into being. In addition to caring for those already ill, social reform and teaching also began its attempts to prevent the healthy from becoming sick and so ultimately child welfare clinics came into being.

Now our hospitals not only care for children medically, but arrange teaching, occupational and play therapy for them and in addition make provision for parents to stay with the child throughout his period of in-patient care. You have chosen an interesting and, rewarding career by joining the staff as a sick children's nurse.

Where Do Our Patients Come From?

Infants and children are admitted to medical paediatric wards for two reasons.

They may have suddenly become ill and have come to hospital as emergency cases and the degree of illness in these cases may vary. Or the children may be admitted to the wards for investigation of symptoms, usually following attendance at an out-patient clinic.

A general medical paediatric ward will contain children of all ages—from small babies to older children approaching puberty.

The severity of their illness is also variable—some may be obviously acutely unwell while others may appear outwardly very healthy.

Usually the atmosphere of the ward is a happy one and although smaller children may appear to be miserable to begin with, few patients do not settle down quite cheerfully.

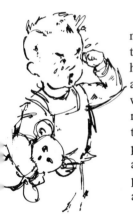

Wise parents and nurses will have seen to it that the child has some familiar and loved 'treasure' with him in this new experience and the other little patients in the ward are the best of all at putting a newcomer at ease.

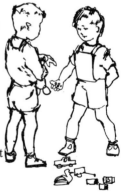

A few minutes spent letting the newcomer meet the children around his bed, exchange of names, etc., is time spent in a valuable way. Equally, explanations as to who the various people around the ward are and what they do is wise.

It is surprising to student nurses how ill a child must sometimes be before he or she shows it and unlike adults who 'dream up' all sorts of symptoms because they feel that this they are expected to do—if a child *feels* well he usually behaves as a well child.

Many adults, when they enter a children's ward, are struck by the noise and movement. Crying may attract their attention more than the joyful sounds—but few patients will be found to cry constantly.

As many patients as are old enough and well enough to be up and about will be playing in the ward as soon as the doctor's morning ward visit is over.

You may find some patients more active than others either because they are fun to be with, good patients, or because their particular condition arouses your sympathy. But you must remember to spread your care and attention widely.

The very quiet child who is 'no bother' may be very worried about being in hospital and will welcome a friendly quiet talk. The deaf child, the blind child, and the mentally retarded child may all tend to be overlooked and overshadowed by the personalities of the more cheerful characters in the ward. But they must all have loving attention.

Although it can be all too easy to form deep attachments with one particular child in most instances this is not wise and may ultimately not be of benefit to the child or to yourself.

Quite frequently children who do not speak English have to be admitted e.g. children who come from foreign lands or those who speak Gaelic or Welsh. Although you may not be able to communicate freely with them through your speech they will be made happier by a friendly face and a friendly tongue. They can be encouraged to play with the other children and active steps should be taken to find if there is in the hospital someone who speaks enough of the child's language to overcome any difficult barrier. Failing this the voluntary workers or men of religion attached to the hospital could be a valuable source of 'language' helpers. There is usually someone in a church who will come forward.

The Child's Parents

Parental attitude to the child and his illness varies a great deal. Some parents whose child has a minor ailment may seem over-concerned; others whose child has a serious illness may appear outwardly indifferent. We must, however, never let our judgement of parental attitude colour our attitude to them. The children belong to them. We are merely given the duty of caring for them during their hospital stay. Remember always that the child will be going back to the home environment from which he came and so we must not do anything to try to undermine that.

Parents will naturally wish to know what is happening to their child and how he is progressing. It is wise for nurse not to enter into deep conversation about the details of his illness and investigations but to refer the parents to discuss such matters with the nurse in charge or to the doctor.

When a child is admitted as an emergency the doctor will usually tell the parents exactly why the child has had to come to hospital, what will happen to the child once he is there, and roughly how long his stay will likely last.

Such a conversation might go thus:-

'Your child has been fevered and unwell these past two days because he has pneumonia. He is not at all well at the moment and will be better with hospital treatment. We are likely to use one of the many antibiotic drugs and this will do him the quickest and most immediate good if it is given by injection to begin with. This can only be done by qualified people who can assess the effect such treatment is having.

In a few days' time he should be much better and his fever should have gone. His chest will be X-rayed at the end of a week and, if the pneumonia has improved, he should be home for you to look after a few days after that'.

In this instance if the parents ask you about the child's progress you can speak only generally about their child's liveliness and improving outlook. Once the course of treatment and the radiological findings are known then you can give a much more accurate and truthful account of what the situation is.

If the child is admitted from a Waiting List for investigations or for a known problem then he may have to have quite a number of tests performed and all the results from these tests collected before a clear reason for his illness can be conveyed to the parents.

Such a conversation might go like this:-

'Johnny has been having diarrhoea on and off for several months now. There are quite a few diseases which may cause diarrhoea and before I can tell you exactly what is wrong with Johnny there are some tests which will have to be done. These tests are done more easily in hospital where the facilities are.

The tests will include several X-rays and blood tests and examinations and may take a week or so to complete.

As soon as I have all the results gathered and have considered them I will speak to you again and tell you exactly why your child has diarrhoea. By that time too I will be able to tell you what we can do about curing the condition for him.

If Johnny's parents were not told about the tests and they came to see him only to discover that he had had a 'special X-ray' that morning they would, with justification be very worried and think there had been some serious turn of events instead of expecting this.

Even as it is the parents are very worried so doctors and nurses should not add to this burden unless there is a sudden unexpected turn of events and even then the parents should be told by some of the professional staff and not be left to find out from Johnny himself!

Doctor and nurse alike must be very careful if any adult does ask a question about a child in the ward that this adult is the parent, next-of-kin, or appointed guardian of the child.

Grandparents, uncles, aunts, friends are all welcome to visit the children (if medical condition of the patient permits it). Confidential information about a patient's progress should not be passed on to any of these unless they are the 'official' person acting for the child.

2

General Aspects of a Medical Ward

You may well find the pace in a medical ward in many ways slower and less dramatic than that in a surgical ward or orthopaedic ward.

Some medical emergencies do need very swift treatment and very close and constant care—a child suffering from status epilepticus or a baby with severe broncho-pneumonia or a poisoned child would require immediate attention at emergency level.

In other instances, and often for the majority of cases in the ward, it will seem that the doctors plod gently round in the morning ordering one or two investigations here and there and then waiting for results.

It is necessary to investigate symptoms and signs before we can prescribe proper treatment and give parents a fair assessment of their child's illness, and the likely progress.

During the waiting time of course the doctor spends time getting to know his patient—and this takes quite a time with some children—and in establishing a good relationship with the child where he is trusted and looked to as the person who will make whatever is wrong better!

Observation is of the Greatest Importance

When a child is admitted to hospital a full medical history is obtained. This is not only an account of the child's present complaint but also of his birth history, and early development; his family and his past history.

Most of the patients cannot inform us what they feel wrong and so we must question the parents carefully to obtain all the facts—even though some may seem irrelevant at the time.

Thereafter we rely upon our own observations a great deal to help us assess progress. The nurse is of particular value here because she is with the child a substantial part of the day. She can tell the doctor a great deal about feeding habits, how and when he vomits, etc.

Temperature, pulse, and respiration rate are usually charted and these yield a lot of useful information about the patient's condition.

3
A Few Points about the Normal Child

Before we can discriminate what is abnormal it is important to know a little about what is normal regarding infants and children.

The Period of Childhood

The period of childhood is divided into sections as this helps to describe the age group of a child.

1 *Perinatal Period*
   This is the period from onset of labour till the end of the first week of life.

2 *Neonatal Period*
   This period is from birth until the end of the first month of life.

3 *Infancy*
   This period is from the end of the first month to the end of the first year of life.

4 *Toddler*
   This period is the years from one to three.

5 *Pre-school Child*
   This period describes the child aged three to five years.

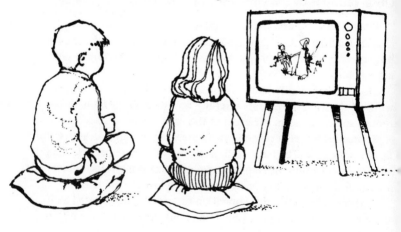

6 *Childhood*

   The fixing of a definite age group to this is rather more difficult
   and usually is reckoned until puberty begins.

7 *Puberty*

   The age of onset of puberty varies greatly. The age range varies
   from ten to fifteen years but is commonly around the twelve to
   thirteen mark.

   Most paediatric wards do not admit children over the age of
   twelve and a half years.

The human infant at birth is physically, intellectually, and
emotionally immature and he depends for a substantial period on the
care of adults around him—especially of his mother.

During his first year he makes relatively greater mental progress
and physical (psychomotor) strides than at any other time in his life
providing he is given warmth, nourishment, rest, and love.

We can assess his psychomotor development by making certain
observations and measurements—some of which are recorded below.
Remember, however, that these are averages and that normal children
can vary widely from them. It is useful to have them as a general
guide, however.

Observations and Measurements

   Weight

   The average British newborn baby weighs about 3.2 Kg. at birth.
During the first six months of life he gains about 0.6 Kg. per month so
that he more than doubles his birth weight in that time.

   During the next six months he gains about 0.5 Kg. per month so
that he has trebled his birth weight by the time he is one year old.

   From the age of one year to five years he gains approximately 2.2 Kg.
each year.

   Height

   The average newborn British baby measures about 50 cms. in length
from the tip of his heel to the crown of his head.

   By about one year he is approximately 75 cms. tall.

   By four years of age he is about 100 cms. tall.

Heart Rate
    At birth this is about 140/minute
    At six months this is about 130/minute
    At one year this is about 125/minute
    At four years this is about 100/minute
    At twelve years this is about 80/minute

Respiratory Rate
    At birth this is about 45/minute
    At six months this is about 35/minute
    At one year this is about 28/minute
    At four years this is about 23/minute
    At twelve years this is about 18/minute

It is quite unnecessary to memorise these figures. Special charts are available in clinics and wards with this information on them when it is necessary to find out more accurately what a child's weight or height should be.

Dentition

The infant's first set of teeth (primary dentition) consists of 20 teeth. The first to appear are the lower central incisors and they usually appear between the fifth and ninth months. All twenty teeth should have erupted by the time the child is two and a half years old.

The secondary dentition (permanent teeth) consists of thirty two teeth. The first to appear are molars which erupt about six years of age. The dentition is completed when the wisdom teeth (third molars) erupt which may not be until seventeen years of age or later.

When the infant is teething he may well have some discomfort, be irritable, and 'not at all like himself'.

However teething has often been blamed as a cause of illness e.g. of fever or convulsions—and this is certainly not the case. It has been said by an authority that the only thing that teething produces is teeth and this is the safest way to regard the process!!!

If a child who is at the teething stage has fever, vomiting, or convulsions you must look for the cause of these conditions.

Motor Development

These are only a few points regarding motor development of the child. Books have been written on this subject alone!!!

The infant and child show motor progress at a variable rate and we must be careful not to call him retarded if he is not as quick as his siblings were, or as the child in the next cot in the ward is.

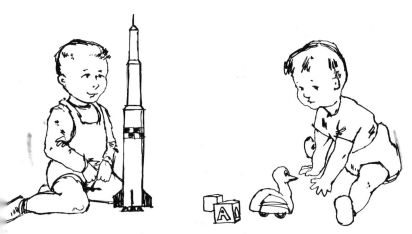

There are many ways of assessing progress but the normal child should be able to do the following things by the ages given:-

2 months	smile and vocalise when spoken to
3 months	support his head strongly when pulled to the sitting position
5 months	lift his head from the pillow
6 months	sit unsupported if put in the sitting position
9 months	sit up by himself
1 year	pull himself up to the standing position and say simple recognisable words
2 years	say simple recognisable phrases
2½ years	have bowel and bladder control

After this stage it is often easier by simple observation to decide if his progress is satisfactory or not.

4
Infant Feeding

Provided he is offered an adequate amount of calories and his fluid intake is sufficient daily, and this is done in a loving and hygienic manner a healthy infant should thrive.

He requires calories for growth, for muscular activity, to allow him to 'tick over', and to replace what he has lost in excretion.

The fat and carbohydrate contents of his food provide most of his energy and the protein builds the tissues.

If the child is allowed about one hundred calories per Kg. of his weight a day he should thrive.

He requires fluid to maintain his hydration, to replace what he loses in urine and faeces, in sweat, and through respiration.

If the child is allowed about 150 mls. per Kg. of his weight per day then his needs should be satisfied.

Remember, however, that there is a great deal of difference in the personal requirements of individual children and common sense must be used along with metric measures!!!

The small infant receives his calories and fluids satisfactorily as milk. The two main ways of providing this are either breast feeding or bottle feeding.

Breast feeding is much less common now than formerly but the choice of feeding method should in most instances be left to the mother. If she chooses not to breast feed then she must not be made to feel inadequate. It does not matter which method is used provided the infant thrives and is happy.

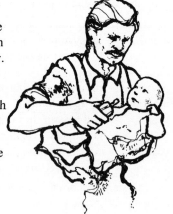

Indeed bottle feeding can include the father much more in the early upbringing of his baby than breast feeding can!!!

The main advantage of breast feeding over bottle feeding is that—providing mother's personal hygiene is good—a breast fed baby is much less likely to suffer from infections—especially gastro-enteritis.

Bottle feeding requires certain utensils and facilities for sterilisation, refrigeration, and for food storage.

If the hygiene of the mother or nurse who prepares feeds is faulty then the feed can easily become infected and the infant may suffer seriously.

There are many proprietary milk preparations. Most of them are based on cow's milk and the product sold as powder or evaporated which is reconstituted by adding water when a feed is being prepared.

Indeed these days firms are even producing already sterilised disposable prepared feeds which only need to be opened and fed to the infant.

Prepared feeds are ready to use and may come in disposable sterilised packs with sterilised teats. There is no need for the food or teat to be handled until it is actually used.

No one preparation is better than another for every baby in spite of what the manufacturers claim in advertising.

A newborn baby is best fed on half-cream preparation. These contain less fat than full cream ones and are probably easier to digest on account of this.

The change to full-cream milk may be made according to the infant's demands and usually by the age of six to eight weeks he will be established on a full-cream preparation.

By the age of about four months or a weight of 5.6 Kg. both breast and bottle fed babies will be taking about 180 ml. each feed with five feeds daily. About this time mixed feeding is introduced. This gives the infant much more varied and interesting diet but it is also of importance in providing him with iron. He requires iron to prevent him from becoming anaemic.

This requirement for iron only manifests itself now as when he was born he had some iron in reserve to use and his milk feeds also provided a little to add to it but by three to four months this supply will be nearly exhausted.

Mixed feeding usually starts with the addition of a small amount of cereal to the diet twice daily. The cereal powder is mixed with some of the measured milk feed but should be fed by spoon and not added to the bottle of milk. Infant cereals high in protein and iron are used.

The amount of cereal is gradually increased—there is no need to use sugar to sweeten it or to tempt him as if he is really hungry he will eat it and not then develop the habit of having too much sugar. Later prepared infant foods with a wide variety of tastes are introduced making visiting relatives, holidays, days out very easy for the mother to organise as far as baby's feeding is concerned.

The baby should continue to have milk feeds from breast or bottle until he is six to nine months old. Many babies indeed can drink quite nicely from a cup long before this stage is reached. Thereafter sterilised cow's milk should be offered to the child.

The gradual introduction of solids into the baby's diet is called weaning.

In addition to the calories, fluid, and iron the infant must be given certain vitamins if he is to grow satisfactorily. The most important of these which we give as supplements are Vitamin C and Vitamin D. Neither of these is contained in adequate quantity in breast milk although most artificial feeds are fortified with Vitamin D and some contain Vitamin C.

Throughout his first year whether he be breast or bottle fed the infant should be given vitamin supplements.

Vitamin C prevents scurvy and is usually given as orange juice or rosehip syrup.

Vitamin D prevents rickets and aids healthy growth of bones and teeth. It used to be given as cod liver oil or Adexolin. Vitavel or Government Vitamin Drops containing both vitamins D and C are best.

By the time the baby is one year old he should drink boiled cow's milk and other fluids and should be taking small helpings of the family's diet where suitable.

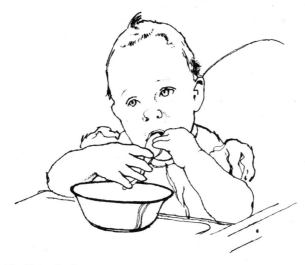

Diet in Hospital

We feel that infants' and childrens' diets in hospital should be prescribed by the doctor.

Some children require very specialised diets as will be seen later. For example for children with diabetes or the infant with phenylketonuria normal diet may be dangerous.

It is wise therefore for nurse not to give any child food until the doctor has prescribed it and particularly important that she should either temporarily prevent relatives bringing food or should intercept any food that they do bring till she is quite sure that the doctor approves and that the nurse in charge knows.

5

Common Investigations

When a child develops symptoms or signs of illness—whether acutely or over a long period—it is the doctor's business to diagnose the reason for these. If he does not make a proper diagnosis then he cannot decide on proper treatment and nursing care.

The doctor is helped to make his diagnosis by three distinct pieces of information which he must gather:-

1 The History

This is the story of the *symptoms*, or what the mother (or child if he is old enough to tell) notices is wrong.

The history is very important because by listening carefully to what the mother says and by asking thoughtful questions the doctor is able to decide in his mind what are the likely reasons for the symptoms in each case.

2 Physical Examination

Once the doctor has heard the history he will perform a routine physical examination of the patient.

He may pay particular attention to the system he feels may be causing the symptoms which have been described but he will also make sure that he examines the patient thoroughly in other aspects as well.

The physical examination will provide him with the *signs* of illness and help to confirm the diagnosis.

3 The Investigations

These are all additional tests or procedures which will help to confirm the diagnosis and also the results may indicate to the doctor how serious the illness may be.

Sometimes only one or two simple procedures are required. Sometimes many tests—simple and complicated—may be required.

N.B.

It must be remembered by the nurse that she too must listen attentively and intelligently if she is around when the history is being taken.

It is not always necessary for a patient to be admitted for investigations. Many tests are performed quite satisfactorily at out-patient clinics or casualty departments. The parent in this case is asked to return again when the results are known or to contact her own practitioner who will have the reported findings at his disposal.

If many or complicated technical tests are required then the patient is usually admitted to hospital during the time required.

Once the diagnosis is reached and confirmed special treatment may be needed and some of the investigations may be repeated at intervals to see if the treatment is having the desired effects.

Some of the tests which require to be done may be painful and uncomfortable for the child. If this is the case the doctor may prescribe sedation for the child.

This has two main advantages:-

1 the child will be asleep during the procedure and should neither feel pain nor remember the discomfort once he is awake again
2 if the child is asleep it is much easier for the doctor and nurse to perform the test since they do not have to contend with a frightened struggling child

Some tests are painful but may be so for a very short time so that using sedation would be rather like using a sledge-hammer to kill a small fly. However, doctor and nurse should never pretend to the child that there will not be pain when there will be. It is always better to be simply truthful, especially when you know the test may have to be repeated at another time. In this instance the child is much less likely to co-operate if you lied to him the first time.

6

Investigations Involving Simple Observation

The nurse by her close and continuous contact with the patients can pass on to the doctor a lot of information from her own observations.

For example if a baby is admitted for investigation of vomiting nurse will be able to observe how and when he vomits, what he vomits, and how well or badly he feeds. Similarly she will be able to tell about the frequency and consistency of stools of a patient with diarrhoea. Although these points seem simple and unimportant they are often of a great deal more value than a string of complicated and uncomfortable tests.

When a child is admitted with convulsions it is you—the nurse—who will be able to describe the type of seizure and how many are occurring and subsequently you will be able to say whether the treatment is being effective or not.

The *weight* and *height* of children and infants are always recorded on their admission to hospital. They are easily performed tests but may give quite a lot of relevant information about illness and progress.

If they are to be of any real value they should be measured carefully and always in the same manner and if possible using the same scales and measuring stick.

If a baby is not thriving well or a child has started a special diet it is often valuable to weigh them every day so that the effect of treatment can be assessed.

There are many other examples you can think of which would on the surface seem basically simple and unimportant but in reality which are of the utmost importance to the doctors working in the wards.

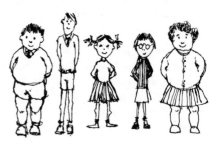

7

Investigations Involving Urinalysis

Urinalysis

Samples of the patient's urine can tell a great deal about illness and progress.

Some tests are so simple to do and so important that urine should be tested routinely at least on admission of the patient.

When there are any abnormalities found a daily urine examination is often indicated.

Simple Tests Include:-

1 *The appearance*

Normal urine may vary in colour from almost clear to orange.

The colour varies with the concentration of different substances present in the urine.

Some urines are clear and some are cloudy.

Abnormal colours include the dark brown of bile-containing urine and the smoky or dark red urine which contains blood.

Occasionally very odd colours—blue or green—occur but this can usually be traced to the child having had highly coloured confections!!!

Occasionally too there is a slight red appearance in urine when a child has been drinking the black currant juice concentrates. It is useful to know if this is the case.

2 *The Specific Gravity*

This is a measure of how concentrated urine is. It is measured by a simple glass instrument called a *hygrometer*.

The hygrometer is put into a jar of urine and it will sink to a varying level according to the concentration, and the specific gravity is read from this point.

The normal range is from about 1002 (weak) i.e. low specific gravity to 1030 or more (concentrated) i.e. high specific gravity.

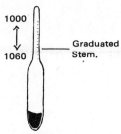

1000 ↕ 1060 — Graduated Stem.

Left: Hygrometer

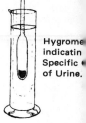

Hygrome indicatin Specific of Urine.

Right: Hygrometer in Jar

The specific gravity depends on how well the kidneys are able to concentrate or dilute the urine. It will be low if the child has been drinking a lot of fluid, it will be high if he has been drinking little or is dehydrated from some other cause, because the kidney will try to preserve as much fluid for the body as it can. When there is chronic renal disease the kidney may become unable to vary the specific gravity at all and then it may be always the same—around 1010.

3 *Abnormal Constituents*

The usual ones which are tested for are:-

> protein
> sugar
> ketones
> blood
> pus

Nowadays the first four are easily detected by 'stick' or tablet tests (Ames) which show colour changes if they are positive. These tests are based on rather complicated chemical tests which may still be used.

Protein

Protein should normally not be detected in the urine. If it is present it may be shown by using Albustix, or by boiling the urine when protein appears as a white cloud when acetic acid is added.

Proteinuria indicates that there is something wrong with the kidney:-

a little may be present in urinary tract infection,

a moderate amount in acute nephritis,

a great deal in nephrotic syndrome.

Sugar

Sugar should not usually be present either. When it is, the sugar is usually glucose and the usual reason is that the child has diabetes mellitus. Sugar may be detected by Clinistix—which simply registers that sugar is present or Clinitest which indicates how much sugar is present.

As well as detecting diabetes mellitus in the first place testing for sugar can tell how satisfactorily the disease is being controlled when insulin therapy starts.

Ketones

Ketones are tested by Acetest or by ferric chloride. Ketones are substances formed in the blood when the child has to break down his body tissues e.g. when he has an illness which makes him eat or drink poorly or when he is not able to use his food and drink properly.

They may occur if the child has a fever and loses his appetite.

They may also occur in untreated diabetes because the child cannot use his food properly having insufficient insulin.

Blood

Blood may be present in large amounts—and the urine appears red—or in microscopic amounts and the urine may appear clear.

Blood appears in the urine in acute nephritis or when there are stones in the renal tract—to mention a few of the many reasons.

Pus

Pus occurs when there is an infection in the renal tract. If there is a lot of pus the urine may appear cloudy white.

N.B.

> The only way to be sure if there is pus or blood in urine is for the specimen to be examined under the microscope.

pH

The *pH* of urine is a measure of how acid or alkaline the urine is. A low pH means acid urine and a high pH means alkaline urine. The pH should vary according to the kidney's response to the body's need for acid or alkaline products.

Twenty-Four Hour Urine Collection

A collection of the total amount of urine passed by a patient in twenty-four hours may be needed for a variety of reasons:-

1 we may simply want to know the quantity of urine being passed-
   he can pass a very large amount in diabetes insipidus and a very
   small amount if his kidneys are failing

2 we may wish the twenty-four hour specimen of urine collected so
   that we can measure how much of a biochemical substance he is
   passing in urine every day

Whatever the reason the result of the test can only be of value if the collection is complete and it may be difficult in the small infant or 'disturbed' child—however, it should not be impossible.

If some urine is lost e.g. if the child wets the bed it may be helpful to assess how much is lost rather than to throw out the collection and start again. In this event the important thing is to tell whoever is in charge of the test what has happened so that they can adjust their calculations accordingly.

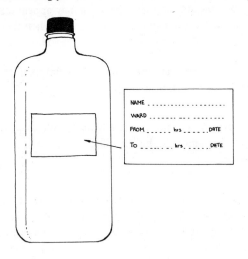

8
Investigations Involving Blood Examination

Blood is usually taken by syringe and needle when a largish volume is required and by skin prick when a small amount will do.

Skin pricks give capillary blood samples and are easy to perform. In the

older child the tip of the thumb is often used and in the baby the heel. Skin prick tests are used for measuring haemoglobin and white blood cell count.

Larger blood samples are usually taken by venepuncture, i.e. puncture of a vein. In the older child there are suitable veins in the elbow region or the back of the hand.

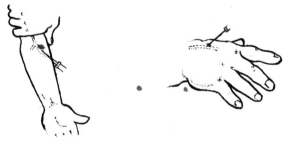

The appropriate part is cleaned with a simple antiseptic like methylated spirit or hibitane then dried with a sterile swab. Nurse may be asked to constrict the arm above the site so that the vein to be punctured becomes engorged and more easily seen. The arm should be constricted by firm rather than tight pressure. Nurse will also need to keep the other arm of the patient well out of the way in case it should hamper the procedure!!!

This form of puncture is usually simple and quick to perform.

In a small infant there are often no veins of a suitable size present in the arm. In such a case blood would have to be taken from a large vein such as the femoral or external jugular vein, or from the sagittal sinus.

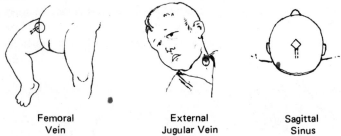

| Femoral Vein | External Jugular Vein | Sagittal Sinus |

The preparation is the same as for simple venepuncture but the nurse will have to hold the child firmly and properly if these procedures are to be straightforward.

The femoral vein is found in the groin. The infant is placed on his back without his nappy and nurse holds his legs firmly down in the abducted position.

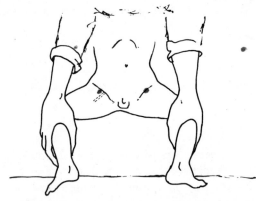

Doctor locates the vein by feeling for the femoral artery pulse. He knows that the vein is right beside this and is guided where to make the puncture.

The external jugular vein is usually easily seen when the infant's neck is turned to the side.

Nurse should wrap the infant in a blanket so that his arms and legs are immobilised. He is then laid on his side with his neck extended over a pillow. This brings the vein well into view.

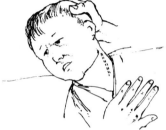

Nurse will hold the infant's head with one hand and the body with the other. Doctor will make a venepuncture in the usual way.

The sagittal sinus is a very large venous channel running centrally along the top of the infant's head. Blood is obtained from it by 'fontanelle tap'. The sagittal sinus can therefore only be tapped in a very small infant whose fontanelle is still open.

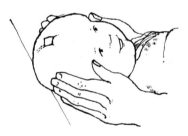

The baby is wrapped in a blanket to control his arms and legs. He is then placed on his back with the back of his head on the edge of the table. If there is a lot of hair on the head the fontanelle area should be shaved. The shaved skin is then cleaned with antiseptic.

The doctor then makes his puncture at the posterior angle of the fontanelle. This procedure sounds a bit alarming but if done carefully is not in the least bit dangerous.

After venous blood is obtained from any site the puncture wound is covered by a sterile swab and firm pressure is exerted on the area *until bleeding stops.*

It is easier to stop bleeding after external jugular or fontanelle tap if pressure is exerted with the infant raised to a sitting position.

The importance of the nurse's role in every one of these procedures can be seen. She is the person who not only helps doctor professionally but she reassures and comforts her little patient as well.

Venous Blood

Venous blood is used for a large variety of examinations including measurement of urea and electrolytes, blood calcium, blood culture—and many more.

E.S.R. (Erythrocyte Sedimentation Rate)

The erythrocyte sedimentation rate is a measure of the rate of fall of the red blood cells in a sample of blood.

It is a most useful investigation in many illnesses.

Normally the red cells would only fall about 10 mm. in one hour. In illness they may fall up to 100 mm. or more in one hour.

The test is of value in assessing the progress of such illnesses as rheumatic fever when in the initial phase the E.S.R. is often very high indeed to begin with but as the child regains health the E.S.R. returns to normal.

It is not very clear why the cells should settle faster in illness than in health but the fact that they do makes this a very useful test.

9
Lumbar Puncture

This procedure is performed when we wish to examine the cerebro-spinal fluid (i.e. the fluid which surrounds the brain and the spinal cord).

The usual reason for examining the cerebro-spinal fluid (C.S.F.) is when meningitis is suspected.

In a small infant or an unconscious child no sedation is usually given. In an older child it is kinder to sedate and our practice is to use a rectal sedation. This is easily given, acts quickly and efficiently and should eliminate pain thus making the procedure simple.

The nurse's important role is once again in careful and firm holding of the child.

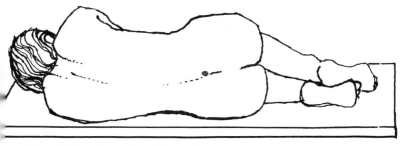

The child is laid on the table usually on his left side in such a way that his back is right at the edge of the table.

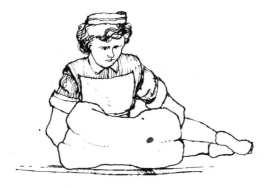

Nurse then flexes his back fully by putting one arm round his neck and one arm round the back of his knees.

Having cleaned the skin area over the lower lumbar spine the doctor will insert the special lumbar puncture needle between the vertebrae until he feels it enter the cerebro-spinal space.

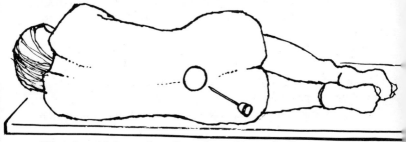

When he withdraws the stilette from the needle fluid should drip

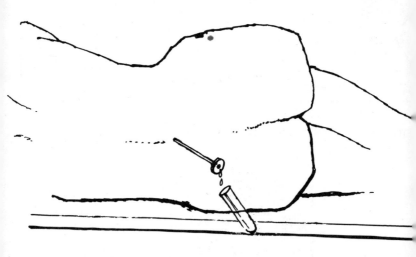

out and may then be collected for examination. (Sometimes the reverse procedure can be employed to administer certain drugs, e.g. for meningitis).

10
X-ray Examinations

These examinations are valuable and are very frequently used.

Straight X-ray

For this there is no special preparation of the child apart from removing any objects which might show on the films!!! (hair grips, badges, etc.). The appropriate part is X-rayed quickly just like taking a photograph. A straight X-ray may be taken for example of the chest in pneumonia, of the abdomen in obstruction, of the wrist in rickets, etc.

Special X-ray Procedures

Special X-ray procedures may require special preparation of the patient and may take longer to complete.

When special preparation for an X-ray is required everyone concerned must be very careful to carry out the radiologist's instructions otherwise time and effort is wasted and indeed the child may be subjected to irradiation with a useless outcome.

Many of these involve the administration of a radio-opaque substance to the child—that is a substance which will show up on the X-ray film.

Such procedures include:-

> (a) barium enema
>   barium meal and follow through
>   barium swallow

These procedures investigate the alimentary tract.
>   and

> (b) intravenous pyelography (I.V.P.)

This procedure outlines the renal tract.

Examples of X-ray Findings

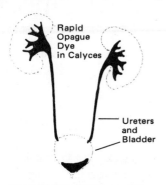

Rapid Opague Dye in Calyces

Ureters and Bladder

Normal I.V.P. (Diagrammatic).

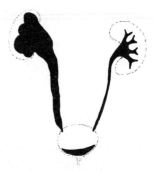

Diagram of I.V.P. appearance with Hydronephrotic Right Kidney and Ureter.

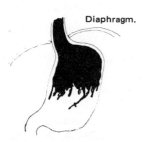

Diaphragm.

Diagram of Barium in normal Stomach.

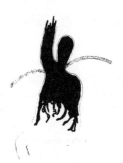

Diagram of Barium outlining Hiatus Hernia.

Summing Up

In concluding this short chapter on procedures to help diagnosis it must be pointed out that those mentioned are only a few of the battery of tests which are now at the disposal of the medical teams.

However, the well-tried simple things frequently give all the information that is required to supplement the observations of the nurse to aid the doctor to complete his diagnosis.

11
Medical Diseases of Children

Medical diseases by and large are those which cannot be put right by operative techniques—as used in surgical disorders and orthopaedics. This does not mean of course, that they cannot be cured, but some will require special drugs and medicines—some for a long time—if the patient is to become healthy.

The reason for a disease is decided according to the symptoms and signs with which it presents. In the following paragraphs some of the illnesses you are likely to meet in a medical paediatric ward are described. This has been done under 'systems'. You will notice that some symptoms occur under several systems, and are not specific to any one disease. This makes history, observation, and careful choice of investigation very important in reaching a proper diagnosis.

Vomiting for instance may be a prominent symptom in many infections (e.g. gastro-enteritis, meningitis, pyelonephritis) and in other illnesses (e.g. pyloric stenosis, hiatus hernia, feeding problems and so on).

Cyanosis may occur in heart disease and respiratory disease.

Oedema may occur in heart disease, kidney disease, and nutritional disorder.

Jaundice may occur in liver disease and blood disorders.

12
Alimentary Diseases

The Alimentary Tract

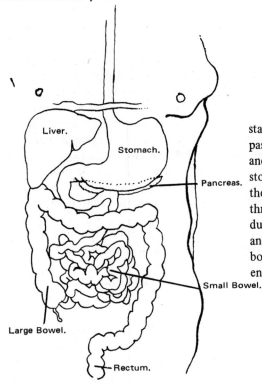

The alimentary tract starts at the mouth, passes down the pharynx and oesophagus into the stomach. Then through the small bowel (its three parts are called duodenum, jejunum, and ileum) into the large bowel (the colon) and ends at the rectum.

Its function is to allow:-

1 ingestion of food
2 mixing and digestion of food
3 the absorption of what the body requires
4 the rejection of what is not required

The Alimentary Tract (contd.)

The waste is of course excreted as faeces.

Digestion is aided by the secretions which certain glands put into the alimentary tract.

The mouth accepts food and therein it should be properly chewed.

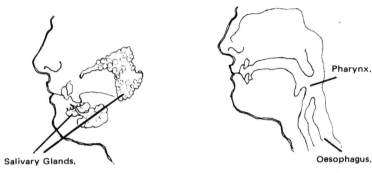

Salivary Glands.

Pharynx.

Oesophagus.

Digestion begins in the mouth with the help of saliva secreted by the salivary glands.

The pharynx and oesophagus are simply passages which lead the food into the stomach.

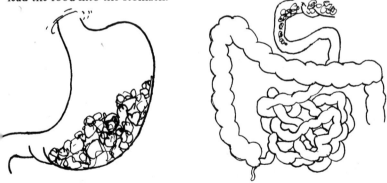

The stomach is the great mixer and its action churns the food into a semi-solid mass which will pass more readily into the small bowel.

Digestion also proceeds in the stomach because the stomach produces hydrochloric acid and other digestive chemicals (enzymes).

The main part of digestion occurs in the upper parts of the small bowel.

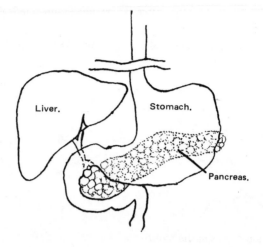

The wall of the small bowel secretes enzymes. Both the liver and the pancreas secrete very concentrated enzymes into the small bowel. As the food passes along it is broken down into very small parts which can easily be absorbed through the gut wall. Most of the absorption takes place in the lower small bowel.

The small food particles resulting from digestion are absorbed through the gut wall into the blood stream and thus pass to the parts of the body which deal with changing them into chemicals which can be used to replace and rebuild tissues as required.

The large bowel absorbs a lot of water as the food residue passes along it. This is important in preserving proper body hydration.

Some alimentary diseases are due to:-

1   upsets in the gut's ability to digest and absorb

2   mechanical faults in the alimentary tract

3   liver or pancreatic disease

4   infection

3

Mechanical Faults

There are two common disorders found in infants which present with vomiting and which are due to upsets in the 'mechanics' of the alimentary tract.

1 Congenital Pyloric Stenosis

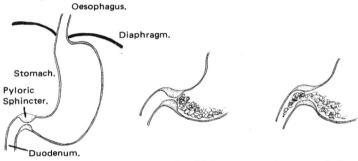

The pyloric sphincter is a muscle which separates the stomach from the duodenum. It opens and closes according to need and allows food to pass gradually from the stomach.

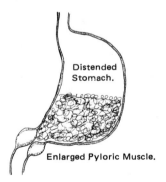

In congenital pyloric stenosis this muscle becomes hypertrophied—much bigger and thicker than usual—and this causes an obstruction at the outlet of the stomach.

The cause of this disorder is not known but it is probably a form of genetic or inherited disease. It most commonly affects boys. It may affect father and son, it may occur in several infants in one family.

Symptoms and Signs

The infant is usually well until he is three or four weeks old and then he begins to vomit. Initially it may be only once or twice a day but then he vomits with every feed. The vomit usually leaves the stomach in a typical forceful manner which we call projectile and it may shoot two or three feet from his mouth. In spite of his vomiting the baby is very keen to feed and always seems hungry. Because of the vomiting he loses weight and becomes scraggy. He also becomes constipated.

The diagnosis is made by 'test feeding'. The infant is sat comfortably in a warm room naked, either on nurse's or mother's knee or on a table so that he can be examined properly. Nurse or mother feeds the infant by bottle or breast according to the baby's upbringing. Doctor feels his abdomen and if there is pyloric stenosis he will feel the pyloric muscle as a lump about the size of his thumb nail, hardening and softening. Sometimes just by looking at the baby's abdomen he may see waves of contraction passing across it as the stomach tries to empty food through the pylorus. This is called 'visible peristalsis'.

Treatment

If the pyloric tumour is felt, then it is cured by operation. The surgeon will make a small incision in the infant's abdomen and then divide the pyloric muscle. Once the operation has been done the infant usually begins to thrive very well indeed.

2 Hiatus Hernia

A hernia is a sac containing a small part of the bowel. You will be most familiar with hernias in the groin region. These are easily seen.

A hiatus hernia is a pouch of part of the stomach which passes up through a small hole in the diaphragm. When a hiatus hernia is present ood can regurgitate into the sac and back up the oesophagus very readily when the stomach contracts.

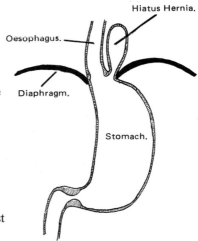

Symptoms and Signs

Vomiting usually starts in the early weeks of life. It may be very frequent but is not so striking as projectile vomiting. The vomiting may contain mucus and altered blood. The infant fails to thrive.

The diagnosis is usually confirmed by a special X-ray test called a 'barium swallow'. While the infant takes a barium feed the radiologist views the oesophagus and stomach on a special screen and will be able to demonstrate the hernia.

Treatment

Propping the infant upright in a 'baby sitter' helps to prevent regurgitation. It is important to keep him upright *all the time* otherwise there is no point in this part of the treatment. There is no use for instance in feeding him propped up and then gaily lying him head down on your knees to change him!!!

Thickening his feeds with cereal also helps to stop regurgitation and so each bottle feed will usually have cereal added.

Because the stomach contents are acid and regurgitation of the acid into the oesophagus may cause scarring and narrowing which may worsen the vomiting an antacid substance is given with every feed.

Most infants on this regime will show improvement and begin to thrive. Once they reach the stage of eating a mixed diet and of sitting up by themselves their symptoms have usually gone completely.

There are other 'mechanical' faults which lead to vomiting most have a surgical cause (bowel obstructions) and so will not be dealt with here.

14
Faults in Digestion

The three major components of our food are:-

1   protein

2   carbohydrate

3   fat

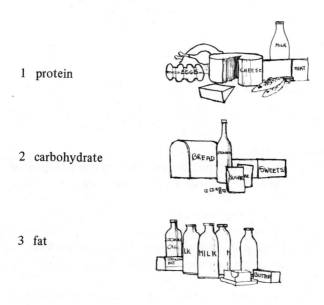

During digestion, special enzymes work on each of these components until they are reduced to particles small enough to be absorbed. The special enzymes are secreted mainly by the small bowel wall, the pancreas and the liver. If these enzymes are not produced adequately then the food is not absorbed properly and much of it is lost in the stools. This leads to the malabsorption syndrome. There are many causes but the symptoms and signs may be similar. Usually there is diarrhoea. Because much fat is in the stools, they are pale, greasy, and foul-smelling. Because so much foodstuff is not absorbed the child fails to thrive. As well as losing the main foodstuffs they often do not absorb iron and so become anaemic.

EXAMPLES OF DISEASES CAUSING MALABSORPTION

Coeliac Disease

This is the commonest cause of malabsorption syndrome in Britain. Children with coeliac disease have intestines which are sensitive to the protein which is contained in wheat (gluten). When they eat any food containing gluten the lining of the small bowel becomes partially destroyed and so cannot secrete its digestive enzymes.

Symptoms and Signs

Coeliac disease does not affect a baby who is only being bottle or breast fed because these feeds do not contain gluten. As soon as solid foods are introduced then he may begin to have diarrhoea and fail to thrive. Most children with coeliac disease come to notice between the ages of one to two years because of failing to grow, they are under height as well as underweight, have diarrhoea and are pale and listless.

They often have very thin limbs with loose wrinkled skin in the groins and armpits. They often have swollen abdomens.

Diagnosis

The best way to confirm the diagnosis is to perform a very specialised test called a 'jejunal biopsy'. In this test a capsule is put into the child's jejunum by passing it through the mouth on a long tube. The capsule contains a small knife and when it is in the jejunum the knife is made to cut a very thin piece of the wall away. The capsule is then drawn back up and the piece of tissue is examined under the microscope.

Treatment

If coeliac disease is confirmed the child is treated by means of a special diet which we call 'gluten free'. No food of any kind which contains gluten is given. A special diet sheet is available to help the mother to know which foods the child should not be given, If the diet is carefully followed the child will soon begin to thrive again. Until they are properly well the patients should also be given oral iron to correct anaemia, and vitamins (especially D) to prevent vitamin deficiency disorders.

2 Fibrocystic Disease of the Pancreas (Cystic Fibrosis)

This is a disease which is inherited in a special way by certain children and several children of a family may be affected. The disease was at first thought to be only a disease of the pancreas which is how the name arose but it is now known to affect many parts of the body. The most important parts are:-

1 the part of the pancreas which secretes digestive juices

2 the glands in the respiratory tract which secrete mucus

The illness may show in different ways according to how severely one or other part is affected.

Symptoms and Signs

a. If the pancreatic digestive juices are deficient then the child develops symptoms and signs of malabsorption.

b. If the mucus glands in the respiratory tract are affected then the child develops increasingly severe respiratory infections. The mucus which is produced by the diseased glands is very sticky and so difficult to cough up. It tends to block off the small airways. The lungs easily become infected so that pneumonia recurs. Eventually the lung tissue becomes full of abscesses and the child's ability to breathe adequately becomes more and more impaired. They become breathless after mild exercise and then breathless even at rest. Eventually they will die of respiratory failure. The organism which most commonly causes pneumonia in this illness is the staphylococcus aureus.

c. A child may have symptoms and signs of both malabsorption syndrome and respiratory disease.

The disease usually presents during the first year of life but may not show until later.

Diagnosis

Two special tests are of value:-

a. We may send a stool to the laboratory for measurement of trypsin. Trypsin is an enzyme produced by the pancreas. In fibrocystic disease there will be much less in the stool than usual.

b. A sweat test may be undertaken. Children with fibrocystic disease have much more sodium and chloride in their sweat than normal children. A sample of sweat is obtained and the laboratory will measure the amount of these substances in it.

Treatment

The child with fibrocystic disease is helped best by:-

a. giving pancreatic enzymes by mouth to make up his deficiency. This helps his digestion to return to normal. In addition we give vitamin supplements to prevent vitamin deficiency.

b. giving antibiotics to help prevent respiratory infections. When he or she has an acute respiratory infection they are often helped by nursing in a tent with humidity.

c. physiotherapy—breathing exercises especially, help to maintain the child's respiratory ability.

Prognosis

This disease is usually fatal in childhood because of the progressive and inevitable damage which is caused to the lungs. With adequate treatment, however, more children are now living into adult life.

15

Some Infections of the Alimentary Tract

1 Oral Thrush

Thrush is a fungal infection which is not uncommon in small babies—especially those who are bottle fed.

Symptoms and Signs

It is recognised by the presence of small white patches on the lining of the baby's mouth. They may look like milk curds but are difficult to scrape off. The baby with thrush has a sore mouth and so finds feeding painful. He may refuse to finish feeds or may cry a lot during feeding and so swallow a lot of air, and vomit.

Treatment

The infection is easily treated by dropping into the mouth a special preparation of Gentian Violet three times a day for three days only. As the infant's teat will also be infected care must be taken not to allow it to come into contact with those of other infants.

2 Acute Stomatitis

This is a very painful infection—probably due to a virus which affects infants and children. The child becomes ill with fever, lost appetite and irritability.

Symptoms and Signs

The mouth and lips become affected by many small ulcers which may readily bleed. Because of the soreness, the child may be very reluctant to feed or drink.

Treatment

There is no special treatment and the infection usually resolves within ten days. The most important nursing feature is to encourage the child to drink and this may be difficult but sometimes the use of drinking straws is rewarding. It is not a very infectious disorder but care should be taken that the child's eating utensils are used only by himself.

3 Gastro-Enteritis

Many different organisms may cause gastro-enteritis and the disease may be very mild or so severe that the infant dies. It usually affects a baby who is artificially fed and if hygiene is adequate should always be avoidable.

Symptoms and Signs

The baby ingests the infecting organism in a feed.

The usual symptoms are the sudden onset of vomiting and diarrhoea, the stools being frequent, watery, and often explosive. According to the severity of the vomiting and diarrhoea, the baby may lose a lot of fluid and quickly become dangerously ill from dehydration.

Treatment

In a mild case stopping all milk feeds and offering the infant clear fluid such as dilute saline for twenty-four hours and then gradually re-introducing milk feeds (graduated feeding) will be sufficient to stop the diarrhoea and alleviate the symptoms. In a severe case the infant will be given nothing orally and its fluid will be administered by intravenous infusion. The intravenous infusion is continued until vomiting and diarrhoea have stopped when a graduated feeding regime is introduced.

Antibiotic therapy is usually given to the severely ill infant to eliminate the infection. The nurse who is looking after an infant with gastro-enteritis must be very careful not to spread the infection. She must be precise about hand-washing and gown wearing at all times.

4 Dysentery

This is another form of intestinal infection due to an organism called Shigella. It may affect a child of any age and again may cause a very mild or very severe illness.

Symptoms and Signs

Usually there will be diarrhoea. The stools usually contain blood and mucus. There may be vomiting. The older child may complain of abdominal pain. Sometimes the infection is so severe that the child develops a high fever and becomes very shocked.

Treatment

Treatment will again vary with severity. Mild cases will usually recover if solid food is withdrawn for twenty-four hours and a liquid diet instituted. A gradual re-introduction of solids is then given. The severely affected child will have to be given fluid by intravenous infusion.

Dysentery is very infectious and barrier nursing is essential if the disease is not to spread.

Antibiotic therapy is usually given to help eliminate the infection.

5 Ulcerative Colitis

This is not a common illness in children but is often a severe one. Its cause is not known. It usually affects the older child and there is often some psychological disturbance which seems to provoke the onset and continuation of the disease. The disease causes ulceration in the large bowel.

Symptoms and Signs

The child begins to have increasingly severe lower abdominal pain and passes very frequent stools containing blood and mucus. The diarrhoea may be very severe so that a lot of weight is lost. The amount of blood lost in the stools may make the child very anaemic.

Diagnosis

The diagnosis is made by examining the mucus lining of the large bowel through a special instrument called a sigmoidoscope. It is also diagnosed often by performing a special X-ray test called a barium enema in which barium is inserted into the rectum and fills the colon and shows a special pattern.

Treatment

When the child is having a lot of pain and diarrhoea, bed-rest and a light diet often helps. Special medicines may be useful. Often, however, the medical treatment is not sufficient to prevent the continued loss of weight and the bloody diarrhoea and an operation to remove the affected part of the large bowel may be needed.

16
Failure to Thrive in Infants

Failure to thrive is not a disease but a symptom and it is a common reason for an infant being admitted to hospital.

The average full-term new born in this country weighs about 3.2 kgm. and should gain about 0.6 kgm. per month during the next six months. An infant who fails to thrive will gain weight much more slowly or will lose weight. When failure to thrive is severe and the baby is less than 75% of his expected weight he is termed *marasmic*. This is a descriptive term and not a diagnosis, so that when such an infant is admitted we must look carefully for a reason for his failing to thrive.

Clinical Appearance

An infant who is thriving satisfactorily looks healthy—he is of good colour and well rounded and he is happy. The infant who fails to thrive is not happy—he cries frequently and looks miserable. He loses his subcutaneous fat and so appears thin, particularly in his face, limbs and chest wall. The skin is often loose and wrinkled especially in his groins and axillae. A marasmic infant is severely wasted and often looks like an 'old man'.

Causes of Failure to Thrive

The commonest reason for an infant not to gain is under-feeding. If he is offered insufficient nourishment then he is quite unable to thrive, even though he is basically a healthy baby who has no serious underlying disease.

Babies who are underfed often vomit and the basic reason for this is often wind.

For the infant to be satisfied, whether he is fed by breast or bottle, he should have 150 mls. of fluid per kgm. of weight per day and 100 calories per kgm. of weight per day. He should finish his feed within twenty minutes or so and have been winded during and at the end of the feed. When he is fed by bottle, the hole in the teat should be large enough for the milk to drip out at a countable rate when the bottle is inverted. During his feeds the bottle should be held in such a way that the teat is always full of milk.

If these points are not attended to the infant may ingest too much wind, vomit, lose his nourishment and fail to thrive—even though he was born whole and healthy.

For instance, when he is offered too few calories, or too little fluid, he will not be satisfied. He will feel hungry sooner than usual and when given his next feed will suck hungrily and probably swallow more air because of this. Often this fills his stomach up so that he may *appear* to be more easily satisfied and in fact not *finish* his bottle. Mother may then be misled into giving him *less* at his next feed and so a vicious circle is set up. Most artificial milks (powder or liquids) should be reconstituted with one measure of milk to each ounce of water. Sometimes a feed is made too dilute so that although he is given the proper amount of fluid, so that he is not thirsty, his calories are insufficient. Sometimes less fluid is put with the milk in the mistaken idea that the concentrated milk will make him grow better but he becomes thirsty. Sometimes he is given the proper proportions of milk and water but in insufficient quantities. So he is not satisfied, ingests wind and vomits.

If the hole in the teat is too small he spends too much effort in sucking—including air—tires easily and so is apparently satisfied. If the hole is too large milk pours into his mouth and he gulps to swallow it, again filling his stomach with wind. If the bottle is held lazily and the teat is half full of milk only, then every time he swallows he ingests air.

If he is allowed to take much more than twenty minutes to his feed both he and mother become tired and his feeding routine is upset.

All the points are very simply remedied by carefully enquiring *how* the infant is fed and once corrected, he should thrive well.

It is important when an infant does not thrive not to blame the milk. Quite commonly we find such infants have started on one product and because they fail to gain have been changed through a whole range of milks. The important point is to find out why and not to blame the milk product.

The above factors which lead to a basically healthy baby failing to gain we often term 'feeding problems' but there are a number of diseases which can cause failure to thrive too. Some are now mentioned briefly and may be more fully described in other sections.

DISEASES WHICH CAUSE FAILURE TO THRIVE

1 Infections

Any infection if severe enough and long-lasting enough may lead to poor weight gain. Oral thrush for instance causes the infant to have a sore mouth so that he feeds poorly. Gastro-enteritis causes diarrhoea so that he loses much of his nourishment in his stools. Respiratory infections make him breathless so that he may be unable to finish a full feed. Urinary tract infection, septicaemia, and other serious infections may make him anorexic too.

2 Alimentary Disorders

Any disease which impairs the infant's ability to absorb his food can lead to poor nutrition. The two commonest such disorders are coeliac disease and fibrocystic disease of the pancreas.

3 Congenital Abnormalities

Some such abnormalities are obvious causes of inability to feed adequately—for instance cleft lip and palate. Hiatus hernia and pyloric stenosis lead to vomiting early in life and usually because of this symptom to ready diagnosis. Congenital heart disease may make the infant breathless so that he cannot feed adequately.

4 Mental Deficiency

An infant who in his early weeks appears to be normal but feeds poorly and disinterestedly may ultimately turn out to be mentally defective and such a reason must be born in mind when failure to thrive is encountered.

5 Other Causes

There are other rarer or less obvious causes of poor weight gain than those listed above.

Management of the Baby failing to Thrive

Before the infant can be treated we must decide which is the reason for his failing to thrive since each condition has its own specific management. Feeding problems should be readily diagnosable and are completely correctable. It is useful for mother to come frequently to the hospital to feed the baby under nursing supervision until she feels confident in her own handling of him. Infections will require specific therapy, primarily with antibiotics, and many of these will resolve completely so that the infant will become healthy again. Some conditions, e.g. pyloric stenosis require single operations for cure. Others such as cleft palate require several operations for alleviation. Coeliac disease and some rare disorders require special diets to be instituted before the infant becomes happy and healthy. This diet may have to be lifelong.

17

Vitamin Deficiency Diseases

Vitamins are substances which are present in certain foodstuffs and which the baby requires in only small amounts to remain healthy. If these amounts are not supplied however, disease may result.

The four commonest vitamins are Vitamins A, the B complex (vitamin B was once thought to be single but is now known to consist of several separate vitamins) C and D. Only deficiency of vitamins C and D commonly cause disease in Britain.

Vitamin D Deficiency

Vitamin D is the vitamin which prevents rickets and is found in foods such as fish liver oils (cod liver oil for example) eggs, butter and margarine. It is also formed in our skins when exposed to sunlight.

Vitamin D is required to help our body absorb calcium. Calcium is required to produce healthy bones and teeth. Without vitamin D the bones do not calcify properly and so they become soft and deformed (Rickets).

Symptoms and Signs

Rickets is usually recognised in the child between one and two years of age because of certain bone deformities:-

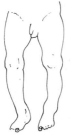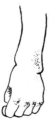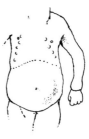

1 bowing of the legs
2 swollen wrists and ankles
3 the chest wall may also be deformed and show a 'ricketty rosary'
4 delayed closure of the anterior fontanelle occurs

Apart from these findings the child with rickets is usually well-nourished and is not ill. It is not a painful disease. The main danger is that if the disorder is not treated the bone deformities become permanent.

Diagnosis

The diagnosis is made by observing the bone deformities. X-rays confirm it because the bones show special changes recognised on X-ray films.

Treatment

Treatment is simply by giving an adequate amount of vitamin D. The child should have 4,000 units daily until rickets is healed.

Rickets will be prevented if the child is given a daily supplement of vitamin D amounting to 400 units. Breast milk and cow's milk do not contain enough vitamin D so that supplements should be given from the early weeks of infancy. Once mixed feeding is introduced the infant obtains some vitamin D in his diet, but it is safer to give vitamin supplements until he is two years old.

The doses of vitamin D mentioned are sufficient for preventing and treating rickets. It is not safe to give too much vitamin D because this may have a poisonous effect on some children.

Vitamin C Deficiency

Vitamin C is contained in fruits and vegetables and prevents scurvy. Vitamin C is necessary for the healthy formation of certain body tissues—especially bones and small blood vessels.

In scurvy the small blood vessels tend to burst readily and so the affected infant bruises very easily. Sometimes bleeding occurs around the bones and this can be very painful. Scurvy is not at all common in British infants because so very little vitamin C is required to prevent it and most infants receive a very adequate amount from orange juice or rose-hip syrup. Vitamin C is not poisonous.

8

Diseases Affecting the Urinary Tract

The Urinary Tract

The two kidneys are important organs whose major function is to modify the amount of fluid and chemicals circulating in the body according to our needs. They do this by secreting urine. A large amount of blood is pumped through each kidney every minute and the kidneys decide how much fluid to retain or secrete and how much of the chemicals should be retained or secreted.

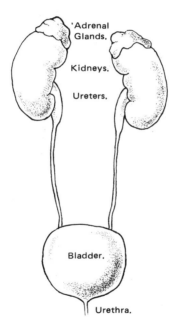

Once the urine is formed it passes from the kidney into each ureter. The ureters are tubes which conduct urine from kidney to bladder. The bladder stores the urine until it is full, when we have the need to empty it by micturating. The urine then passes along the urethra and is execreted.

19
Some Common Diseases of the Renal Tract

1 Pyelonephritis

This means infection of the urinary tract. The infection usually at least affects the kidney tissue and may be present in ureters and bladder as well. Pyelonephritis is common in children (girls more than boys) and may affect any age group from the very small infant to the well-grown child.

The illness may be mild or may make the patient acutely ill.

Symptoms and Signs

There may be a sudden acute illness or there may be less acute but long standing symptoms. Usually there is fever. The fever may be very high and the child may present because of a convulsion. The infant may refuse feeds and vomit. He may become quickly ill and dehydrated. The older child may be able to complain of abdominal pain and pain on passing urine (dysuria). Often they pass small amounts of urine very frequently. Sometimes the urine may smell infected and may look bloody. A child who has been successfully toilet trained and who then begins bed-wetting may be suffering from pyelonephritis.

Diagnosis

Pyelonephritis is confirmed by examining the urine. When there is infection the urine contains albumin and pus, and under the microscope blood is often seen.

To find out which organism is causing the infection and also which antibiotic will most successfully eliminate the infection a specimen of urine is sent to the laboratory for culture. The specimen has to be collected carefully so that infection is not introduced to the urine.

Usually, in a small infant, it is obtained by cleaning up the genital area with a sterile solution and putting on a polythene bag or more scientifically by bladder puncture with a needle. The older child will often co-operate in passing urine and after he has been specially cleaned a

ecimen is obtained from the 'middle' of his excretion, i.e. discarding
ae first urine passed and obtaining the middle part in a sterile
ontainer—a 'mid-stream' specimen of urine (M.S.S.U.).

Treatment

When the child is ill with fever and vomiting he needs rest in bed
nd lots of fluid to drink. Following laboratory findings the appropriate
ntibiotic is prescribed.

Intravenous Pyelogram (I.V.P.)

We are not certain how the urinary tract becomes infected.
ometimes the urinary tract has been formed in an abnormal way, we
now that this often leads to pyelonephritis. Therefore when ever the
hild with pyelonephritis is well enough we perform a special X-ray
est called an intravenous pyelogram (I.V.P.).

Some of the abnormalities may require operation if the infection is
ver to be cured.

Not all cases of pyelonephritis have abnormal urinary tracts. The
najority are perfectly normal. Once the urine contains no pus and the
nfection is controlled by appropriate antibiotic treatment the child
nay go home. Because the infection may readily return the child
hould have antibiotic therapy for at least six months to try to
prevent recurrence.

2 Acute Nephritis

This illness usually affects children of school age. It is associated
with infection by an organism called the B-haemolytic streptococcus.

Symptoms and Signs

Usually there is a history of sore throat, which resolves satisfactorily
about three weeks before the onset of nephritis. Then the child may
become vaguely unwell with headache and perhaps vomiting. Often
oedema—swelling especially of the face and ankles due to excess fluid
in these tissues—develops. The most striking feature is the passing of
bloody urine (haematuria). Examination of the urine shows it to
contain protein. On microscopy we see a lot of blood and a special
feature called 'casts'. A throat swab may grow the B-haemolytic
streptococcus.

Treatment

The child should initially have rest in bed. The reason for his oedema is partly that the diseased kidney is not able to make as much urine as normally, so that fluid is retained in the body. If we measure the amount of urine the child passes in twenty-four hours, it will be found to be less than normal.

Until the kidneys are able to make urine satisfactorily again we restrict the amount of fluid the child may drink. Once the oedema has gone he may drink normally again. The best way to determine this is to weigh the child every day—he will lose weight as he loses oedema until he is back to normal.

Penicillin is usually given by mouth to eliminate the streptococcus.

Most children with this condition recover completely within a few weeks. Blood and protein disappear from the urine. Sometimes the child may be very ill. The degree of illness depending on how severely the kidneys are affected and therefore on how impaired is their ability to work normally.

The Nephrotic Syndrome

A syndrome is a collection of symptoms and signs which commonly occur together. In the nephrotic syndrome the three features are:-

1 gross oedema
2 gross proteinuria
3 the finding of a very low amount of albumin in the bloodstream

There are several causes of this syndrome but in the syndrome as it occurs in children, the cause is not known.

Symptoms and Signs

The syndrome usually presents first in a child of pre-school age. The child becomes vaguely unwell and then develops oedema quite rapidly. The oedema affects the face, the legs and the abdomen. It may be so gross that the child cannot open his eyes. The abdomen may become very distended because of ascites (fluid in the peritoneal cavity).

The reason for the oedema is that the diseased kidneys are not ble to secrete fluid adequately or to retain protein and so protein is lost in large amounts in the urine (proteinuria). A normal amount of protein is necessary in the bloodstream if fluid is to be drawn back from the tissues adequately.

Observations and Treatment

The child is kept in bed until the oedema resolves. He is given a special diet which contains:-

1 a lot of protein to replace that which is being lost in the urine
2 little salt because too much salt in this condition tends to worsen the oedema
3 the amount of fluid he is allowed to drink is also restricted to begin with
4 a special type of drug called a steroid is given and this usually helps the oedema to resolve, at least during the first attack

Within about ten to twelve days the oedema fluid begins to disappear and the child begins to pass a great volume of urine—this is called the period of diuresis. The child should be weighed daily. His weight will be found to fall greatly during diuresis and then weight loss will cease. Proteinuria will also lessen during the period of diuresis. The urine is examined daily for protein content, and its volume carefully measured.

Most cases of nephrotic syndrome will resolve completely but some recur frequently and some of these children will spend a large amount of their life in and around hospital.

Renal Failure

Certain diseases affect the kidneys so severely that they can hardly function at all, and so the patient develops renal failure.

Renal failure can happen suddenly—when it is called *acute* renal failure. There are many reasons for this and many may be cured if treated early and satisfactorily. Renal failure may occur slowly because of long-standing disease when it is called *chronic* renal failure. This cannot be cured satisfactorily, but can be alleviated by special treatment.

20
Disorders of the Cardiovascular System

The Cardiovascular System

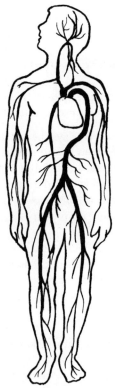

The cardiovascular system consists of the heart and blood vessels. The heart is a hollow muscular pump situated almost centrally in the chest. Its job is to pump blood to all parts of the body.

Schematic Diagram Showing the Heart in its central position with large Blood Vessels coursing to and from it.

The heart is divided into a right and left side, each containing two chambers:-

1　an atrium or collecting part
2　a ventricle or main pumping part

The veins of the body collect the 'used' or de-oxygenated blood from the different parts of the body. As the veins approach the heart they join into the two largest veins called the venae cavae. They pour their blood into the right atrium. It pours the blood into the right ventricle. The right ventricle then pumps it through the pulmonary arteries into the lungs.

In the lungs the blood gives up carbon dioxide, which is breathed out, and takes up oxygen so that it becomes 'oxygenated'. Blood then returns from the lungs along the pulmonary veins into the left atrium which passes it on into the left ventricle. The left ventricle is the most muscular part of the heart and it pumps the blood out into the aorta— the largest artery in the body. The aorta branches into smaller arteries so that oxygenated blood is distributed throughout the body.

To ensure that blood will pass in one direction only there are four important valves in the heart:-

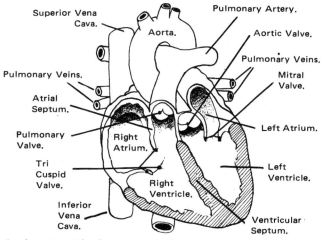

1 the tricuspid valve separates the right atrium from the right ventricle
2 the pulmonary valve separates the right ventricle from the pulmonary arteries
3 the mitral valve separates the left atrium from the left ventricle
4 the aortic valve separates the left ventricle from the aorta

HEART DISEASE

Heart disease may be diagnosed because of certain symptoms, or may be discovered purely by chance.

Symptoms of Heart Disease

1 Cyanosis

The development of a bluish colouration of the skin and mucous membranes. It may occur soon after the baby is born or not until the child is older. It may only occur with exercise and the child may be a normal pink colour at rest. Cyanosis occurs in diseases other than heart disease but is especially common in some forms of congenital heart disease.

2 Breathlessness

This may only occur with exercise, for instance running in the older child, or feeding and crying in the baby. It may be present even when the child is at rest.

3 Failure to Thrive

An infant or child may not grow at the normal rate because of heart disease.

Signs of Heart Disease

1 Cyanosis and Breathlessness

The doctor and nurse may notice these when they are so mild that the parents have not observed them.

2 Finger Clubbing

This is an odd sign which is very common in cyanotic congenital heart disease. The exact reason for it is not known, but the sign is present when the finger (and often toe) nails become rounded and wider than normal

3 The Finding of a Heart Murmur

When the doctor listens to the patient's heart he may hear a murmur. A heart murmur is a sound or noise which should not normally be heard. Not all murmurs, however, mean that the heart is diseased and many normal children and adults may have murmurs which mean nothing serious.

4 The Pulse

The doctor is able to determine quite a lot of information from the type of pulse and its rate.

5 Development of Heart Failure

Certain signs when they occur together indicate that the child's heart is failing.

a. breathlessness at rest (and especially on feeding in an infant)

b. the presence of oedema (swelling of the tissues due to excess of fluid) especially around the eyes, on the hands and feet

c. the finding of a big liver (hepatomegaly)

d. tachycardia—a very rapid heart rate

Many of these signs may occur separately but if they are found together then they usually indicate heart failure.

Heart disease in children is of mainly two types:-

1   Congenital Heart Disease

2   Acquired Heart Disease

1 Congenital Heart Disease

This is the commonest type of heart disease found in children. It can be mild or severe. It may be diagnosed because of the onset of symptoms (as described above)—and the more severe it is, the earlier the symptoms will occur so that sometimes even newly born babies may be found to have congenital heart disease—or it may only be diagnosed by chance—usually because a heart murmur is heard when the child is being examined for some other reason, e.g. when he has a cold, or at a school medical examination.

It is usual to divide congenital heart disease into two large groups:-

> Cyanotic if cyanosis is present
> Acyanotic if cyanosis is absent

Cyanotic Congenital Heart Disease

This type usually presents early in life because cyanosis is an alarming sign to the parents. If cyanosis is present it means that the de-oxygenated blood (which is darker or 'blue') must be mixing with the oxygenated blood (which is 'red'). Cyanotic heart disorders are often very complicated, and quite frequently cause heart failure or failure to thrive.

Acyanotic Congenital Heart Disease

This type may present at any age. Often there are no symptoms and the murmur is heard by chance. Acyanotic congenital heart disorders are not usually complicated. They include holes in the wall (or septum) within the heart which divides it into its four chambers.

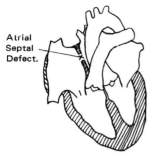

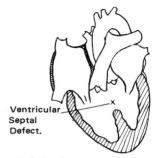

1 a hole in the septum between the two atria is called an atrial septal defect.

2 a hole in the septum between the two ventricles is called a ventricular septal defect.

Sometimes the pulmonary or aortic valves are narrowed (or stenosed) producing:-

1 pulmonary stenosis
2 aortic stenosis

Sometimes a blood vessel called the ductus arteriosus which is required for the circulation of blood in the unborn infant and which should close down once he is born, fails to do so and this produces a common defect called a patent ductus arterious.

Diagnosis of Congenital Heart Disease

The clinical examination of the heart and pulses often leads the doctor to the diagnosis. He is helped by a chest X-ray which shows the shape and size of the heart and by an electro-cardiogram which also helps to tell the size of the heart.

Sometimes special heart investigation has to be carried out to find out exactly what is wrong with the heart and how severe it is.

Treatment

Many congenital heart defects do not require any treatment. Some do require surgical operations if the child is to lead a full and healthy life. The operation may be able to completely correct the disorder and this is usually so in acyanotic congenital lesions. Sometimes, however, the disorder is so complicated that no operation could correct it, but an operation may be performed to help the child at least for a while. This is often so in cyanotic congenital lesions.

When we think a heart murmur means *no* heart disease or only a very minor disorder it is very important that the parents understand that and treat the child in *every way* normally, otherwise the child himself may become over worried about his heart. Even a cyanosed child should be allowed to be as normal as he possibly can—they often know their own limitations much better than their parents.

2 Acquired Heart Disease

The commonest form of acquired heart disease in children is that caused by rheumatic fever. Rheumatic fever is associated with infection by the haemolytic streptococcus.

Symptoms and Signs

The usual story is that the child, who will be of school age, has a sore throat which resolves normally. Some two or three weeks later he develops features of general illness such as fever, loss of appetite and lethargy and typically also painful swelling of the large joints such as the knees and elbows, which tends to flit from joint to joint. He may also develop nodules—small hard lumps on the bony parts of his body such as the elbow, knees, knuckles and skull. A reddish linear rash which comes and goes very quickly called erythema marginatum may also occur. The heart is not always affected in rheumatic fever but when it is there may be an enlargement of the heart and the appearance of a murmur. Sometimes if the heart is seriously affected heart failure occurs. Sometimes chorea occurs. In chorea the child develops bizarre movements of his limbs and face. He cannot help them and they are often described as purposeless. His handwriting deteriorates and he becomes clumsy. The movements are worsened by anxiety. Chorea is much less common nowadays.

Treatment

Treatment of rheumatic fever consists of bed rest, especially when the heart is affected and where there is chorea. Penicillin is given to get rid of the streptococcus and is usually maintained for many years to make sure no further infection occurs. Further infection with the streptococcus may cause more heart damage. Aspirin is usually given for six weeks. It relieves the joint pains and fever. The E.S.R. is raised at the beginning of the illness but should return to normal within four to six weeks and this, together with the resolution of other abnormal clinical findings help to indicate when the child may begin to be active again.

If rheumatic fever is recognised and treated adequately and early it should resolve without leaving the heart damaged. Sometimes, however, the disease affects the heart valves and distorts them. The effect of this may not become evident until the child is grown up when he may develop breathlessness on exertion, or even heart failure.

Upsets of Heart Rhythm

The heart rate is usually regular. It is faster in the infant than in the grown child.

Tachycardia means a faster than normal heart rate. The commonest type of tachycardia is a regular countable rate—perhaps up to 180 beats per min. which occurs with exercise, with fear, or with fever. Once the initiating factor has resolved the heart rate will return to normal.

In some children the pulse may seem to be irregular in that it increases as the child breathes in and decreases as he breathes out. This is called sinus arrhythmia. It is common and of no serious significance.

In infants a condition known as paroxysmal tachycardia sometimes occurs. In this the tachycardia is very fast—usually uncountable—and may be over 300 per minute. It is called paroxysmal because it occurs in episodes between which the rate is normal and the infant is well. During a paroxysm, however, he becomes very ill, may be pale, cyanosed, and breathless. If the paroxysm goes on for long he develops heart failure.

Heart Failure

In addition to paroxysmal tachycardia heart failure may be caused in infants by congenital heart disease and in older children by congenital heart disease, rheumatic fever, and acute nephritis.

Symptoms and Signs

The patient becomes breathless on exercise, feeding, or even at rest. They are usually cyanosed. Oedema, hepatomegaly, and tachycardia are almost constant features.

Treatment

No matter what the cause the therapy follows a standard pattern. Bed rest in a propped up position relieves some of the distress: oxygen may be required until the heart failure is controlled. The most valuable drug for the condition is digoxin. The drug is given in a specific dose for the weight of the child, usually four times on the first day and then twice daily thereafter.

If digoxin alone is not effective a diuretic drug may be added. A diuretic drug acts by making the kidneys excrete more fluid. Diuretics tend to make the body lose potassium in the urine so that potassium often has to be given by mouth to rectify this.

Digoxin is a very useful drug but care must be taken that the correct dose is administered otherwise the child may readily be poisoned by it. Signs of poisoning include vomiting and slowing or irregularity of the pulse rate.

Some causes of heart failure, such as rheumatic fever, will resolve and digoxin may be stopped eventually.

Sometimes as in congenital heart disease, it may have to be used for a long time.

21
Blood Disorders

Blood consists of two parts:

1 The fluid portion is called plasma. Plasma contains some important proteins including those which help the blood to clot. It is also the fluid which carries many substances to and from various parts of the body. For instance—it:-

   a. carries the products of digestion which have been absorbed from the intestine
   b. carries hormones from glands such as the thyroid and adrenal so that they can act on the tissues
   c. carries the electrolytes such as sodium, potassium and chloride which help to maintain the correct composition of the tissue fluids

The number of substances borne by the plasma are too numerous to mention but you can liken it to a busy city street—with people of all types hurrying about their business, one a bank clerk, one a postman, one a housewife and so on.

2 The other part of the blood consists of the cells. The blood cells are of three main types:-

   a. The red cells, or erythrocytes, contain haemoglobin (Hb) whose main function is to combine with oxygen and take it to the tissues, and exchange it there for carbon dioxide. Haemoglobin contains iron
   b. The white cells or leucocytes are of two main types—lymphocytes and polymorphonuclear leucocytes—both of which are mainly concerned with protecting the body against infection
   c. The third type are the platelets, which are not true cells. Their function is to help the blood to clot

The red blood cells, most of the white cells and the platelets are made in the bone marrow—the soft substance contained in the centre of bones. Some of the lymphocytes are also made in the lymph nodes. When the red cells and white cells have reached a certain age they are removed from the circulation, usually by the spleen, the liver and the lymph nodes, and destroyed.

1 Anaemia

When a patient is anaemic his haemoglobin level is lower than normal. An infant's haemoglobin may be normal about 12 gm per 100 mls of blood, the older child's haemoglobin is usually about 14 gm per 100 mls of blood.

Symptoms and Signs

The symptoms and signs of anaemia usually include increasing pallor and increasing tiredness. Sometimes the spleen and liver enlarge. The diagnosis of anaemia is made by finding a low Hb. Examination of a blood film often helps to indicate the cause too.

Treatment

Most anaemias due to iron deficiency will respond to treatment with iron, usually given by mouth but sometimes given by intramuscular injection. If there is an underlying cause such as coeliac disease then it should be treated too.

A patient may become anaemic if:-

a. He loses blood. This may be a lot of blood as may occur in a haemorrhage. Sometimes an ulcer may bleed very slowly so that the blood loss is not obvious and it may be passed out in the stools. In this way he becomes slowly anaemic.

b. He does not have enough iron to make a satisfactory amount of haemoglobin. This happens if a child's diet is low in iron when he will develop a nutritional anaemia.

Nutritional Anaemia in Infants and Children

The newborn infant has a high haemoglobin—perhaps 16-17 gm per 100 ml of blood. For about the first three months of his life his bone marrow does not make a great deal of blood and so his Hb falls over this period to about 10 gm per 100 ml. During his first three months of course he is being milk fed only and whether this is breast or bottle milk his diet during this time will not contain much iron.

When mixed feeding is introduced he begins to be able to absorb some iron and so his Hb will not drop further.

One of the commonest reasons for nutritional anaemia in the first year is lack of iron in the diet and this occurs if there is delay in introducing mixed feeding or if his solid diet contains little 'iron-containing' food.

A child with malabsorption, such as coeliac disease, will not absorb iron and may also become anaemic. Babies with hiatus hernia sometimes lose blood from the mucosa in their oesophagus which may be ulcerated by acid regurgitation from the stomach and so the child becomes slowly anaemic.

    c. The red blood cells are broken down too quickly—a process known as haemolysis. Haemolytic anaemia is not unknown in children but is not common.

    d. The marrow fails to make sufficient red blood cells. This is called aplastic anaemia.

Aplastic Anaemia

Aplastic anaemia is not common in childhood but is a serious, often fatal, disease. Often we find no cause for it. The bone marrow stops making cells of any kind so that as well as becoming anaemic the patient has many fewer than normal white cells and platelets and, so is readily infected, and may bruise easily.

Diagnosis

The diagnosis is made by performing a bone marrow puncture and examining the marrow under a microscope.

Treatment

Treatment includes the giving of blood and platelet transfusions and protecting the child from infection. Steroid drugs sometimes stimulate the marrow to work again but often it fails ever to do so.

2 Purpura

Symptoms and Signs

Purpura describes a finding not uncommon in children. A rash appears. The rash consists of purplish areas due to bleeding into the skin. The areas are usually small. Purpura develops either:-

1 if there are too few platelets in the blood stream
2 the walls of the very fine blood vessels, called capillaries, are diseased

If the platelets are very low then as well as purpura the child may develop very large bruises, often seemingly without reason, or he may have profuse nose bleeds.

3 Idiopathic Thrombocytopenic Purpura (I.T.P.)

This is not an uncommon disease in children. Idiopathic means that the cause is unknown. Thrombocytopenic means a reduced number of platelets and purpura indicates the typical rash.

Symptoms and Signs

It usually occurs suddenly and may follow a respiratory infection:-

1 The purpuric rash may be mild or very florid
2 Sometimes bleeding occurs internally and may be fatal
3 Sometimes nose bleeding (epistaxis) is long-standing and worrying

However, usually the child is quite well apart from his purpura.

Diagnosis

The diagnosis is confirmed by finding a much lower than normal platelet count, without any other abnormality in the blood cells.

Treatment

The attack usually clears up without special treatment and does not recur. If the purpura has persisted many weeks, or if there are so few platelets that serious haemorrhage is a danger, steroid drugs are used and usually cause the platelet numbers to return to normal. Very occasionally it is recommended that the spleen be removed. The spleen seems to be responsible in some cases for destroying platelets faster than normal.

Purpura due to low platelets sometimes happens in other diseases, the commonest being acute leukaemia (see page 71).

4 Henoch-Schonlein Purpura

In this form of purpura the platelet count is normal but there is disease of the capillary walls. Again the cause is not known but it often follows a streptococcal throat infection and is sometimes called allergic purpura. It mostly affects school age children and is not common in infants.

Symptoms and Signs

The rash in Henoch-Schonlein purpura typically appears on the back of the feet and on the knees, ankles, elbows, forearms and on the buttocks.

The rash may be the only evidence of the illness and the child may be perfectly well. Sometimes other symptoms and signs are present including:-

1 painful swelling of joints
2 abdominal pain which may be severe with associated vomiting and even intestinal obstruction
3 haematuria if the kidneys are affected

Treatment

Penicillin is given if the illness is associated with the streptococcus. If there is much joint pain and/or abdominal pain rest in bed and analgesic drugs will be ordered. If there is much vomiting the child may have to have fluids by intravenous infusion.

If there is haematuria then the child has a form of acute nephritis and will require treatment by special diet. The illness may clear up quickly or may come and go for many weeks. It should eventually clear completely.

5 Haemophilia

This is a disorder of the blood-clotting mechanism. Blood-clotting is a very complicated procedure requiring the presence of a number of substances one of which is a protein called anti-haemophilic globulin. The haemophilic child lacks this and so his blood clotting is defective.

Haemophilia is a familial disorder which only affects males. It usually shows in an infant who is learning to walk. When he falls he bruises or bleeds more severely than is expected for the normal tumbles of his age. Sometimes he develops nose bleeds or internal bleeding.

The older boy frequently bleeds into his joints and may eventually become crippled as a result.

Diagnosis

The diagnosis is confirmed by taking a blood sample and finding anti-haemophilic globulin absent or very low in amount.

Treatment

Avoid injury as much as possible. Obviously this means that the boy will lead a very restricted life. When bleeding occurs the only way to stop it is to give him anti-haemophilic globulin which can be prepared from whole blood. Usually it is given as 'fresh frozen plasma' or cryoprecipitate, by the intravenous route. Sometimes many doses must be given. When joints are affected in addition to fresh frozen plasma splinting is often required.

22

Malignant Diseases of Children

Malignant diseases are not uncommon in childhood. Indeed since antibiotics have rendered infections such as pneumonia so readily curable, malignant disease becomes a major cause of death.

Certain tumours may be curable if they are discovered early. Some will not be cured and death will be inevitable even though therapy may prolong life for a substantial period.

Children with malignancy often spend a lot of time in hospital and frequently are admitted when their days are ending because this is easier for the family especially when there are other children at home. In these instances the nurses will become closely involved with a very sick child and with very emotional parents and they will require to be very sympathetic and thoughtful.

Only the commoner malignant diseases will be described.

1 Acute Leukaemia

This is the commonest malignancy in childhood. Leukaemia is a disorder of the white blood cells, usually the lymphocyte as in acute lymphoblastic leukaemia, but sometimes other white blood cells. The cause of the disease is not known. It may affect any age of child but commonly presents in the pre-school years.

In leukaemia the white cells do not mature normally and the immature cells grow in profusion and invade the bone marrow, lymph nodes, spleen and liver. Invasion of the bone marrow means that the normal cells in the marrow cannot grow so that the child becomes anaemic and develops purpura. Invasion of the lymph nodes, liver and spleen cause them to become enlarged and clinically palpable.

Symptoms and Signs

The illness seems to occur quite suddenly. The child becomes progressively paler and more lethargic—may develop purpura, may bruise severely and may bleed very readily. The lymph nodes in the neck, axillae and groins may grow very large and the liver and spleen may become so big as to make the abdomen distended.

Diagnosis

The diagnosis is strongly suspected by this clinical picture. It is confirmed by looking at the blood picture including the Hb, white cells and platelet counts and by looking at the white cells on a blood film. More important is the examination of the bone marrow obtained by bone marrow puncture where the leukaemic cells will be found in abundance.

Treatment

Treatment is not curative but may cause the disease to disappear (a remission) for periods of months or even years and during remission the child will seem a normal healthy child. After a period, however, the disease recurs (relapses) and eventually treatment will produce no remission and the child dies.

Treatment consists of two main parts:-

1 The Use of Drugs
   These include:-
a. steroid drugs which are very effective in producing remission and
b. a group of drugs known as cytotoxic agents. Some cytotoxic drugs are given by mouth but some have to be given by intravenous injection
2 Supportive Therapy
   This includes blood and platelet transfusions when the child is in relapse and the use of measures to protect the child from infection

Present day drugs have prolonged the length of remissions in leukaemia but no cure is yet available.

2 Brain Tumours

Brain tumours are also common in children. They may appear at any age, including infancy. Sometimes they grow slowly, sometimes rapidly. They produce symptoms and signs partly by causing increased pressure within the skull (raised intra-cranial pressure) and partly by their effect on parts of the brain or the nerves themselves.

72

Symptoms and Signs

a. *Due to Raised Intra-Cranial Pressure*

The usual symptoms are of headache and vomiting which worsen as the tumour grows. These symptoms are of course common in childhood for many other reasons but must always be taken seriously until a cause is found.

The signs include papilloedema—this is a swelling of the optic nerve which is readily seen by examining the eye with an ophthalmoscope.

An X-ray of the skull may show 'starting' of suture lines. The 'suture lines' are the lines between the bones of the skull. If there is raised intra-cranial pressure this causes wide separation of these lines.

b. *Due to the Effect of the Tumour on the Brain or Nerves*

There are certain nerves arising directly from the brain which supply parts of the head such as the muscles of the face and eyes. A tumour may damage these so that the child develops a squint or facial paralysis.

The tumour may grow in a part of the brain supplying the arms or legs so that they may become paralysed.

A common site for a brain tumour is the cerebellum which is concerned with maintaining balance. A tumour here may cause staggering and falling, clumsiness with fine movements such as writing and an odd movement of the eyes called nystagmus.

Diagnosis

The history of symptoms and the finding of the above signs indicate strongly the possibility of a brain tumour. Confirmation is by special tests performed by neurosurgeons.

Treatment

If possible the surgeon will remove the tumour completely but sometimes its situation makes removal impossible. Radiotherapy may be given with effect together with surgery, or on its own. Cure of brain tumours is possible, but the outlook is usually grim.

3 Neuroblastoma

This tumour arises in a part of the nervous system called the sympathetic system —this part controls functions of which we are unaware, such as bowel peristalsis, as opposed to those of which we are aware such as limb movements. It may also arise in the centre of the adrenal gland.

It is a very malignant tumour and spreads very readily to other parts of the body such as the liver, skull and bones. In spite of this it is one tumour which occasionally disappears spontaneously.

Symptoms and Signs

If it presents in a young infant the usual features are of failure to thrive and marked enlargement of the liver. The older child may present with bone pains, abdominal swelling or signs of raised intra-cranial pressure.

Diagnosis

The diagnosis is confirmed by examining tissue from the tumour (a biopsy) or sometimes by examining the bone marrow.

Treatment

This consists of the use of radiotherapy and cytotoxic drugs, and the surgical removal of the tumour if possible. The outlook is much better in the small infant, but must usually be regarded as grim.

4 Nephroblastoma

This is a tumour of the kidney, usually occurring in the pre-school age. It readily spreads from the kidney to other parts of the body— especially the lungs. It presents more commonly by the large swelling produced by the tumour being noticed by the parents. The diagnosis may be confirmed by special kidney X-ray (I.V.P.).

Treatment

Treatment is by surgical removal which may be curative if the tumour is discovered early enough. Radio-therapy and cytotoxic drugs are also of value, but again the outlook is difficult to predict.

23
Diseases of the Respiratory System

The Respiratory System

The respiratory systems consists of the two lungs and the system of airways leading to them. Its function is to allow the exchange of oxygen into and carbon dioxide out of the blood stream. Respiration is the process by which air is moved in and out of the lungs.

The airways include the nose and mouth, pharynx, larynx, trachea, bronchi, and bronchioles. Their function is to lead air into and out from the lungs. The lungs themselves consist of innumerable very small sacs called alveoli. In the walls of the alveoli are fine blood vessels called capillaries. The walls of the alveoli are so thin that oxygen readily passes into the blood in the capillaries. It becomes re-oxygenated. The carbon dioxide, which is a waste gas produced by the tissues, readily passes out of the blood into the alveoli and can be expired.

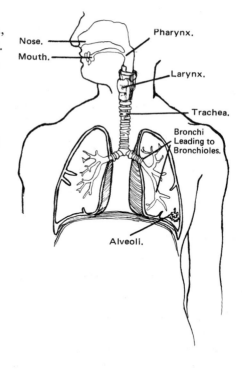

Nose.
Mouth.
Pharynx.
Larynx.
Trachea.
Bronchi Leading to Bronchioles.
Alveoli.

The most common disorders of the respiratory system in infants and children are acute infections. They are conveniently divided into:-

1 those of the upper respiratory tract (U.R.I's).
2 those of the lower respiratory tract.

ACUTE INFECTIONS OF THE UPPER RESPIRATORY TRACT

The upper respiratory tract consists of the airways from the nose down to the end of the bronchi. Infections may affect any one part in particular or several parts in general. They are usually caused by viruses but may be caused by bacteria. They vary in severity but certain symptoms and signs are common to them all.

Symptoms and Signs

Often the onset is sudden. The patient develops fever, irritability and loss of appetite. They may develop a nasal discharge and cough and may complain of a sore throat. On examination they appear flushed. The temperature may rise very high even in a minor upper respiratory infection. After a day or two, even if cough and nasal discharge seems worse, the fever often settles. The patient then regains his appetite and normal good cheer. Febrile convulsions commonly occur at the onset of acute U.R.I's.

1 Acute Rhinitis

This is the correct name for the common cold and it is very common in young patients. It will cause a variable degree of illness but is not usually dangerous.

Symptoms and Signs

The prime symptom is a nasal discharge which may be watery or purulent.

Management of Small Babies

In a small baby a cold may be more troublesome if it causes much nasal blockage. A small baby requires his nose in order to breathe.— His mouth is used for feeding. Obviously if his nose is blocked he may have a lot of diffculty in breathing and feeding at the same time. He may therefore have to be fed more slowly with frequent stops. Sometimes the nose may be gently cleaned with cotton wool pledgets. Occasionally we use special nose drops for a day or two if the discharge is very thick.

2 Acute Tonsillitis

Symptoms and Signs

Here the main symptoms will be of sore throat. There may be pain on swallowing and there may be enlargement of the neck glands (lymph nodes).

Diagnosis

On examination the tonsils are large and inflammed and may have pus on them.

Treatment

Most cases of tonsillitis will be viral and will get better by themselves. Some, however, will be due to the bacteria called streptococcus and in these cases penicillin is usually given to make sure this infection is eradicated.

3 Acute Bronchitis

Symptoms and Signs

The infection mainly affects the bronchi. The child may be quite ill with bronchitis. As well as fever he often has a dry cough, an audible wheeze, and breathlessness.

Treatment

Antibiotic therapy is usually given and the patient may benefit from being nursed in a tent with humidity.

Management of Child

Although most upper respiratory infections are not serious and will not usually require much specific therapy it is well to remember that the infected child often does not feel hungry. Not eating will do no harm, but the child must be offered adequate fluids or he may become quite dehydrated.

4 Croup

Croup is the name given to infections of the larynx which result in a crowing sound (croup). The commonest reason nowadays is acute viral laryngitis.

Symptoms and Signs

Like other 'U.R.T.' infections the onset is acute and the degree of illness is variable.

Management of Child

The child will benefit from nursing in a humid atmosphere.

5 Acute Laryngeo-Tracheo-Bronchitis

This is a very serious infection which affects infants and small children. It is probably a viral infection and it causes inflammation of the larynx, trachea and large bronchi.

Symptoms and Signs

It may start as a milder infection with fever, cough and perhaps some wheeze. The patient rapidly becomes more ill. Because of the inflammation a great deal of mucus is secreted. This blocks the airways. The child has difficulty in moving air in and out of his lungs. He becomes more and more breathless and cyanosed. He usually becomes exhausted with the effort he has to make to breathe.

Management of Child

These children require very careful nursing. They usually require to be nursed in oxygen and high humidity and may have to be tube fed. Sometimes the infection is so severe that a tracheostomy (an operation in which a small hole is made in the trachea into which a tube is inserted) is performed. This helps to make breathing easier and also helps to make suction of mucus out of the airways easier. In spite of this operation, however, the illness is very dangerous and unfortunately may end in death.

6 Asthma

Asthma occurs frequently in childhood. It may affect a child from his early years. The asthmatic attack may be provoked by infection but also seems to be associated in some patients with allergy to substances such as pollen or animal fur or feathers or house dust. Psychological upset may also stimulate an attack.

Symptoms and Signs

Clinically the attack usually begins suddenly and the main feature is the onset of wheezing. Wheezing is due to broncho-spasm (spasm of the muscles in the wall of the bronchi). This spasm causes the bronchi to narrow and makes during respiration the movement of air in, and especially out, difficult. The child becomes frightened, breathless, and may be cyanosed.

Occasionally the attack may be so severe or so prolonged that a dangerous situation, called status asthmaticus ensues.

Treatment

The acute episode may be stopped by the use of a broncho-dilating drug which relieves the spasm of the bronchial muscle. Some of these drugs may be given orally. If the episode is more severe adrenaline is injected sub-cutaneously and this is usually more effective. In status asthmaticus if standard broncho-dilating drugs in repeated dosage are not helpful, steroids may be used.

Management of Child

Nursing in oxygen and humidity may also be indicated.

It is important that the attendant nursing and medical staff do not panic. Calm handling of the situation will be very beneficial to the child.

Once the acute attack has passed, if the child is old enough, deep breathing exercises may prove of value in relieving or lessening the severity of future attacks.

Otitis Media

This is an infection of the middle (or inner) part of the ear and is mentioned here because it commonly occurs with respiratory infections—especially of the upper tract. It may occur at any age and may affect both ears.

Symptoms and Signs

The child is usually fevered and may be acutely ill. The infection causes pain which the older child can tell of but the infant may indicate by pulling or poking at his ear, or rolling or banging his head.

Diagnosis

The diagnosis is made by looking into the ear and seeing an inflammed, bulging ear drum. If the infection is not treated then the ear drum may peforate and pus may discharge from it.

Treatment

The administration of an antibiotic—usually penicillin—by intramuscular injection, is effective. As in other acute infections care must be taken to ensure that the child has plenty to drink. Before antibiotics were available, the infection often spread to affect part of the skull called the mastoid, producing mastoiditis, but this should rarely happen nowadays.

24
Infections of the Lower Respiratory Tract

In infants two diseases of the lower respiratory tract are common. Chest X-ray is a very helpful investigation in determining the extent of these and their progress.

1 Acute Bronchiolitis

This is common in the winter months. It is a viral infection and the inflammation primarily affects the bronchioles.

Symptoms and Signs

The illness may occur suddenly or may follow two or three days after an upper respiratory infection. The infant becomes progressively more breathless and agitated and may be cyanosed. Breathing is obviously an effort and he develops indrawing of his ribs and a harsh wheezy cough. The more respiratory difficulty he has, the more anorexic he becomes. Maintaining adequate hydration may be a serious problem. There is usually no pyrexia with acute bronchiolitis.

Treatment

Most infants will require nursing in a humid atmosphere and many will also require high oxygen concentration too. If they are very ill, antibiotics are usually given. If the infant can feed orally he should be allowed to, but he may require smaller frequent feeds. Sometimes he will have to be tube fed.

The illness may last several days before it begins to resolve and though it may be severe for some time, recovery is the rule.

2 Bronchopneumonia

In pneumonia there is infection of the alveoli. In infants it tends to be patchy but widespread so that many parts of the lungs are affected. The usual cause is infection with the staphylococcus.

Symptoms and Signs

There may be a preceding upper respiratory infection. The infant then becomes ill with fever, anorexia, breathlessness and often cyanosis. He may have a distressing cough.

Treatment

Treatment consists of administering antibiotics to combat the infection. Nursing in humidity and oxygen when cough and cyanosis are severe. Tube feeding may be required. Most infants will recover completely. Occasionally in staphylococcal pneumonia an abscess forms in the lung and this may rupture into the pleural cavity (the space between the lung and the chest wall). If much pus collects in this space we have an empyema and the pus may have to be removed by inserting a needle and drawing it off into a syringe.

3 Lobar Pneumonia

In older children pneumonia is more likely to affect only one lobe of a lung—*lobar pneumonia.* The infection is usually due to the pneumococcus but may be viral.

Symptoms and Signs

The illness usually starts suddenly with fever, general unwellness and cough and there may be pain in the chest. The child is often flushed and apprehensive as breathing causes pain. Clinical examination will usually reveal signs of pneumonia and a chest X-ray will confirm it and indicate its extent.

Treatment

Penicillin by intra-muscular injection is usually quickly effective. Rest in bed, often propped up, will help to relieve pain, but sometimes an analgesic drug may be needed. Attention must be made to ensure that the patient has an adequate fluid intake. Recovery nowadays is usually complete.

4 Tuberculosis

This infection has diminished in frequency over the past few years partly because of:-

1 the effect of present day antibiotic drugs.
2 the earlier detection of infectious cases by mass radiography.
3 the use of B.C.G. vaccination in protecting the child against the infection.

Tuberculosis is a chronic infection due to the tubercle bacillus. There are two main types:-

1 the human bacillus.
2 the bovine bacillus.

The bovine bacillus used to commonly cause infection through milk contamination but Britain now has tuberculosis-free milk herds and this source of infection is now extinct.

Children are now affected through contact with an adult who has active tuberculosis. They usually obtain the infection by inhaling the bacillus so that the usual site of initial infection is in the lungs.

The infection is initially called 'primary'. When a child has a primary tuberculosis infection he may not even be aware of it as the body may deal successfully with the infection so that no symptoms occur.

Symptoms and Signs

If symptoms or signs occur they happen about six weeks after the infection is contacted and may be:-

a. development of a rash called erythema nodosum. This usually appears on the legs and consists of painful red lumps. There are other reasons for erythema nodosum but most are due to tuberculosis.

b. development of a form of conjunctivitis.

c. development of chest pain (pleurisy) with a pleural effusion.

d. development of rather vague symptoms such as fever, loss of appetite. loss of energy, weight loss. Cough may occur but it is not a common feature and the child does not produce sputum with primary tuberculosis.

Diagnosis

The diagnosis is suspected by the above findings and is confirmed by performing a skin test for sensitivity to tuberculosis called the Mantoux test. This consists of a small injection of specially prepared tuberculin material into the skin. If the child has tuberculosis the Mantoux reaction becomes strongly positive showing as an inflamed and sometimes blistered area.

A chest X-ray is usually done and may show evidence of the primary infection.

When a child has tuberculosis we often perform an early morning (before breakfast) gastric lavage on three successive days and send the washings to the bacteriology laboratory for culture.

The child will not cough up the organisms in sputum for culture as an adult will, but mucus from his chest will be swallowed into the stomach especially overnight so that the organism may be grown from the washings.

Treatment

This consists mainly of giving anti-tuberculous drugs. Some are given by mouth, others by intra-muscular injection. Treatment in primary tuberculosis is usually for at least six months. Initially the patient may have to be kept in bed, and indeed may wish to be, but usually he rapidly becomes well enough to be up and about. Providing conditions are satisfactory much of his treatment may be given at home.

5 Post-Primary Tuberculosis

If the body fails to deal with the primary infection itself, and if the condition is not then recognised and treated, post-primary tuberculosis may occur. Two main ways are likely:-

  1 The primary infection spreads through the lungs producing a tuberculous bronchopneumonia.

Symptoms and Signs

The child becomes progressively more ill with fever, weight loss, loss of appetite and usually develops a cough and breathlessness. There are usually physical signs of pneumonia and the chest X-ray will also show it. The Mantoux test will be positive.

2 The infection may gain access to the blood stream and spread to other parts of the body.

a. Meninges

One of the earliest and most dangerous site of spread is to the meninges—the covering of the brain and spinal cord—producing tuberculous meningitis.

Symptoms and Signs

This may also start gradually with loss of appetite, weight loss and fever but then headaches and vomiting occur. If the diagnosis is not made the child may become unconscious, may develop convulsions, paralysis of his limbs and even blindness. He will have neck stiffness and the infant may have a bulging fontanelle.

Diagnosis

The diagnosis of meningitis is made by performing a lumbar puncture and finding an increased number of white cells in the fluid. The infecting organism may be grown from the fluid. In the child with tuberculous meningitis the Mantoux should be positive.

b. Kidneys

When the infection spreads through the blood stream, tuberculosis may occur in the bowels, joints, and kidneys, but it often takes very many months for signs and symptoms to develop in these parts.

Treatment

Treatment of post-primary tuberculosis will be by administering drugs which will be used for up to eighteen months.

The child with primary tuberculosis is not usually infectious to other children and may be treated in a general ward. The child with post-primary tuberculosis may be infectious and may have to be isolated for therapy initially.

Tuberculosis if detected early should not now be fatal but if post-primary tuberculosis develops than some permanent damage to affected organs may result.

Stridor

Croup is one cause of a symptom called stridor. Stridor refers to a particular noise made by the child during respiration. It always means that there is some obstruction in the laryngeal or tracheal areas. As well as acute infections stridor may be caused by a foreign body such as a peanut or small toy which the child inhales, or by diseases causing pressure on the larynx—for example certain tumours.

25

Disorders of the Nervous System

The central nervous system comprises:-

1 the brain (the cerebral hemispheres and cerebellum) within the skull. The cerebral hemispheres contain the highest centres of control and awareness and each part of the body has a 'patch' allotted on the hemisphere. The right hemisphere controls the left side of the body and vice versa. The cerebellum is primarily concerned with balance. The cranial nerves include those concerned with smell, vision, eye movements, facial movement and sensation, hearing and those connected with the heart and lungs.

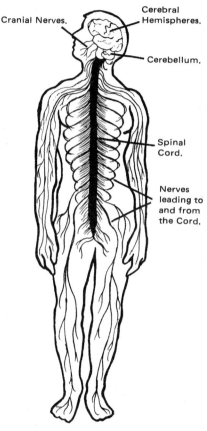

2 the spinal cord within the vertebral column and the nerves leading to and from the cord (spinal nerves) or brain directly (cranial nerves).

The nerves consist of two main types:-

a sensory nerves which convey sensation—pain, touch, temperature, position and so on.

b motor which supply muscles and allow actions to take place.

The nerves are connected via the spinal cord with the brain: some of their activities are automatic and we are not conscious of them but by their connections to 'higher centres' not only do we become conscious of them but are able to actively control them.

Disorders of the nervous system can be complicated. Only the most common disorders will be considered.

1 Mental Deficiency

This term indicates that the mind has failed to develop completely. Mental deficiency may be of mild degree so that the child may be educated at a school for the mentally sub-normal, or so severe that the child merely vegetates. There are very numerous causes but they may be divided into two big groups:-

a. *Congenital Causes*

In this group the infant is destined to be mentally subnormal from the time of conception, because there is something wrong with the genes, or genetic make up. The best known in this group is the mongol child.

b. *Acquired Causes*

In this group the baby at conception is destined to be normal but something then happens to cause retardation of mental development. This might happen before the baby is born, for instance if the mother has a severe haemorrhage so that the baby may not receive enough oxygen, or if the mother has certain infections such as German measles (rubella). It may happen at the time the infant is born. If he is asphyxiated at birth for any reason so that he fails to breathe for some time then the brain may be damaged. It may happen at any time after birth, for instance if the child has severe uncontrolled convulsions, or contracts encephalitis.

These disorders need not lead to mental deficiency of course, but may do so.

Symptoms and Signs

How do we recognise mental deficiency? In some instances it is obvious. We know for instance that no matter how cheerful and sociable a mongol child may be, he is mentally defective. In other instances we have to assess the child's ability at different ages and compare his ability with the average ability for that age. To help in this we often refer to psychomotor milestones. During his first two or three years the child makes great physical and mental strides so that he changes from being a completely helpless and dependent newborn whose abilities are little more than to breathe, feed, excrete, and cry to a determined, enquiring and individual personality able to do a great deal for himself. He makes the biggest strides during his first year.

Whilst by no means complete the list of some of the psychomotor milestones which are useful in assessing an infants progress can be helpful (see page 11).

a. By eight weeks he should smile and vocalise and should be able to follow objects.

b. By twelve weeks he is able to hold his head steady when pulled up to sitting and will turn his head to sound and movement.

c. By six months he is able to maintain a steady sitting position without support, if sat up, and will grasp objects offered.

d. By one year he should pull himself up to standing and say a few recognisable short words.

e. By eighteen months he should be walking unsupported and can make simple verbal commands.

f. By two and a half years he should have bowel and bladder control by day and night.

It is much easier to assess a child's progress after the infant period than before. It is important not to label him retarded if he is 'slow' in only one or two features, however, and it is better to observe him over several months to be certain rather than cause intense anxiety by suggesting that he may be retarded.

Some children who are mentally retarded indulge in odd or repetitive behaviour such as head banging or rolling, hand regard, and teeth grinding. An infant who is either 'very good' or who cries incessantly for no reason may ultimately turn out to be retarded. Convulsions are common amongst retarded children, but of course do not always indicate mental retardation.

What to Do for the Retarded Child

There is no specific treatment to cure mental retardation. In some instances careful management, e.g. at birth or during diseases later acquired—may avoid the development of mental retardation. In two relatively common conditions—cretinism and phenylketonuria—retardation may occur if they are not recognised and treated early. Apart from these two there is no specific therapy. Sedative drugs and anti-convulsant drugs may help the parents to manage a retarded child. Some children will be educable or trainable to some degree but many will be too severely retarded. In these, placement in an institution is usually necessary sooner or later, and is often of importance for the secure health of the rest of the family, especially where the presence and demands of the retarded child mean some neglect of normal siblings.

Cretinism

The thyroid gland is situated in the neck. It secretes hormones which are essential to normal growth—especially of the brain and bones—and for maintaining body metabolism. In cretinism the infant either is born without a thyroid gland, or with such a small gland that the supply of hormones becomes insufficient for normal growth.

Symptoms and Signs

Signs of cretinism become more severe as the infant grows. He usually has a dull, disinterested face. Often a large protruding tongue. Frequently an umbilical hernia. He develops a cold dry skin, sparse hair; and while he may be plump, is always dwarfed. His cry may be hoarse. He may feed very poorly. If the early signs are not recognised

d he is not treated then he becomes progressively more mentally
tarded. This is the most serious effect of cretinism.

Treatment

Treatment consists of giving the cretin thyroid hormone usually
powder or tablets. The starting dose is small but gradually built
up until the signs are reversed. If too much thyroid hormone is given
en the effects of overdose, including tachycardia, sweating, excitability
d hyperthermia, become evident. Once the correct dosage for the
ild has been ascertained he must continue on therapy all his life.

Goitrous Cretinism

Sometimes the thyroid gland makes an imperfect thyroid hormone—
e which does not have the normal actions. In its effort to supply the
dy adequately with hormones the thyroid gland enlarges producing
goitre' in the neck. This is a very important feature in these cretins.

Treatment

The treatment is as outlined above.

26
Convulsions

Convulsions are common in childhood. There are several different types.

1 Grand Mal Seizures

These are the commonest form.

Symptoms and Signs

In this type, the onset is sudden with loss of consciousness and rhythmic jerkings of the limbs and face. Often all limbs are affected but the fit may only involve one side of the body. The child may become cyanosed and increased salivation may be apparent. The fit may last for a few seconds and cease spontaneously or may go on for many minutes.

There may be a passage of urine and faeces during the fit. After it has stopped the child may sleep for a period—the 'post-ictal' phase. Sometimes the limbs may be temporarily paralysed following the fit.

There are many causes for grand mal seizures. The commonest in childhood is a febrile illness—usually an upper respiratory infection, otitis media, urinary infection, or a specific infection such as measles or chickenpox. Febrile convulsions are frequent in children between the age of one and two years: often they cease spontaneously, and they usually occur at the beginning of the febrile illness.

Treatment

There are two lines of treatment to be employed. Firstly general therapy which includes careful positioning of the child so that he does not injure himself during the fit and so that he does not inhale vomit or excretions. When necessary suction of secretions from the nose and throat should be done. Certain anti-convulsant drugs are used by intra-muscular injection to stop the convulsion at the time. Once the seizure is under control the doctor will try to find if there has been

y specific reason for it, e.g. fever—and give specific therapy for this
it is indicated. When fever is high tepid sponging is useful, sometimes
th cool fanning.

The second line of therapy is the use of anti-convulsant drugs to try
control further seizures. They are not routinely used in simple febrile
izures but may be in other situations causing grand mal seizures.
ombinations of these drugs may have to be adjusted frequently to
otain good control of seizures. If after a period of two years no
rther seizures have occurred, and are not likely to recur, anti-
onsulsant therapy may be withdrawn.

Petit Mal Seizures

These are very brief seizures in which the child has a momentary
ss of consciousness: there is no twitching or cyanosis but they may
e very frequent. The electro-encephalogram (E.E.G.) or tracing of the
rain's electricity activity, usually shows a specific pattern in petit mal.

Treatment

These are usually also treated with drugs.

Infantile Spasms

These seizures occur in infants and usually start about the age of
ive to six months. Other names for them are lightning seizures or
alaam fits and these are descriptive terms. The fits are very swift but
usually occur in long runs, perhaps of twenty or more. The infant may
ry out at the onset and then he suddenly jerks his head forward and
lexes his limbs. Although they tend to occur in a baby who has been
developing normally, they almost always lead to mental deficiency. In
his type of seizure the E.E.G. is again very helpful.

Treatment

The only treatment which seems effective in stopping these seizures is a
course of A.C.T.H. by intra-muscular injection: lasting usually for four to
six weeks. It is not by any means always successful so that the fit may continue
unabated making the likelihood of mental retardation much stronger.

27
Meningitis

This is the commonest infection of the nervous system. The meninges are the coverings of the brain and spinal cord and in meningitis they become infected and inflammed. In addition to tuberculous meningitis which has been mentioned and which is now much less common in this country, there are two main types of meningitis:-

a. pyogenic—in which the cause is a bacterial infection such as meningococcus, pneumococcus coliform or haemophilus influenzae and

b. aseptic meningitis which is due to virus infection.

Symptoms and Signs

The symptoms and signs of both are in many ways similar except that aseptic meningitis is less severe and is rare in infants.

The child with meningitis is fevered, irritable, anorexic and has headache. Vomiting is frequent and convulsions may occur.

The important signs are those of neck stiffness and, in the infant, bulging of the anterior fontanelle. When the meningococcus is the infecting organism the child often develops a purpuric rash and may rapidly become very seriously ill and collapsed.

Diagnosis

The diagnosis is confirmed by performing a lumbar puncture to examine cerebro-spinal fluid and finding an increase in the number of white blood cells therein. Normally there should be less than five per c.mm. In pyogenic meningitis there may be several thousand. The C.S.F. is examined also to determine the infecting organism.

Treatment

In pyogenic meningitis treatment with antibiotics should start at once. There are different antibiotic combinations for different causes.

The child may also require intravenous fluid or gavage feeding until he feels well enough to drink and feed orally again.

Providing the diagnosis is not long delayed and treatment is prompt and efficient the outlook in pyogenic meningitis nowadays should be good.

Viral or aseptic meningitis is also confirmed by lumbar puncture but the C.S.F. will have only a moderately raised white cell count and the culture will be sterile. There is no specific therapy other than supportive and the illness should resolve completely.

28
Cerebral Palsy

This is a condition with a number of causes which is common in children. Whatever the cause, damage is done to the brain at some stage in its development. The damage done is permanent but does not progress, and usually manifests by abnormalities of movement. Many children with cerebral palsy are in addition mentally defective but this is *not* a necessary feature.

The causes of the condition are very much those mentioned with mental deficiency and include pre-natal brain damage as well as pre-natal and post-natal causes. In many instances no cause is apparent.

Symptoms and Signs

Children with cerebral palsy have often been referred to as 'spastics'. This is because the commonest resulting disorder of movement is spasticity of the limbs. Spastic limbs are stiff limbs. All the limbs may be affected (a spastic quadriplegia) or the limbs on one side of the body only may be affected. Although spasticity is the commonest disorder, the limbs may be flaccid or lacking in tone, or the child may show athetosis (slow writhing movements of the limbs). Speech is often affected too.

Diagnosis

This usually becomes apparent as the infant grows and his milestones are delayed and abnormal movements develop. If he is severely affected this may be apparent in the early weeks of life. We find evidence of abnormal limb tone and the persistence of reflex actions which should disappear in the early weeks.

Treatment

As the condition is non-progressive no therapy will prevent it worsening, but the degree of brain damage may be severe so that many aspects of normal brain function may be affected. These include the child's motor ability with reference to locomotion, intellectual ability, and speech, hearing and sight. The earlier the diagnosis is firmly made the better will his management be. Some children may have normal intellect but severe physical handicap and so may have to have special schooling in a school for the cerebral palsied: some will have severe mental and physical defect and may require institutionalisation. Proper management may involve co-operation between the paediatrician orthopaedic surgeon, physiotherapist, speech therapist, hearing specialists and eye specialists.

29
Diabetes Mellitus

Insulin is a hormone produced in the islet cells of the pancreas. In diabetes mellitus there is either insufficient production of insulin or the insulin produced is destroyed before it can have its desired effect.

Insulin is essential for normal carbohydrate metabolism and to enable the body to use glucose. In its absence the body is unable to use glucose which builds up in the blood stream and is excreted in the urine. Glucose is a source of energy and if the body cannot use it, then it breaks down other tissues to use them.

Symptoms and Signs

Diabetes mellitus is often familial. It frequently has a fairly acute onset in children. Over a period of three or four weeks sometimes the child may develop thirst, polyuria, polydipsia, an increased appetite and weight loss. If the diagnosis is not made, and therapy instituted, at this point, then the child may become severely ill.

As the blood sugar rises and the body uses more and more alternative sources of energy the child becomes more dehydrated, vomiting supervenes and the child may lapse into coma. In this severe stage of the illness he will appear very ill—sunken, dehydrated and with a poor peripheral circulation. He also develops a specific type of breathing, known as acidotic respiration, characterised by deep, pauseless cycles. His breath may smell sweet due to acetone.

Diagnosis

The diagnosis is made by the finding of glycosuria and acetonuria, glucose being present at about 2% level in the urine. The blood sugar will be greatly raised.

Treatment

When the child is dehydrated and vomiting, intravenous fluids are required to rehydrate him. Insulin is administered, usually by intra-muscular and intra-venous injection initially. The amount of insulin required is judged and adjusted according to the initial blood sugar level and the rate of clearing of glycosuria.

Once he is rehydrated and vomiting has stopped the child may begin to eat again. The diet is usually adjusted to restrict the amount of carbohydrate ingested and high content carbohydrate foods such as sweets, cakes etc. must be avoided. The diet must contain sufficient calories to allow the child normal growth and energy. The insulin dosage is adjusted to try to maintain his urine sugar free or at least below 1%. Insulin has to be given daily and must be given by injection. This part of treatment may lead to family difficulties in management. However, once stabilised, the child should lead as normal a life as possible.

A diabetic child should always carry a card saying so and a glucose tablet in case he feels unwell because of hypoglycaemia.

During stabilisation it sometimes happens that the blood sugar is brought too low—producing hypoglycaemia. This is a dangerous condition which may produce convulsions and brain damage if not recognised and treated. The signs include lethargy and sweating, a full bounding pulse and gradual unconsciousness. Treatment is to administer glucose—by mouth if the child is conscious, by gastric tube if not conscious or by intra-venous injection given by doctor.

It is particularly important that children should be encouraged to manage their own tests etc. to maintain their independence.

30
Jaundice

The yellow colour of the skin and conjunctivae which is present in jaundice is due to an excess of the chemical substance bilirubin in the circulation. Bilirubin is formed when red blood cells are broken down: as this happens to every red cell after its life of one hundred and twenty days or so, there is always a little bilirubin in the blood stream but in jaundice the amount increases greatly.

Formation of Bilirubin

Red blood cells contain haemoglobin: when they are broken down the haemoglobin is separated into two parts—globin, a protein, which is kept in the body—and haem. Haem is a complex substance which contains iron: during its breakdown the iron is conserved to form more haemoglobin and the rest of the substance forms bilirubin. This bilirubin has not yet reached the liver and is called 'indirect' bilirubin: indirect bilirubin can dissolve easily in fats but not easily in water. Indirect bilirubin is taken to the liver and this organ converts it into 'direct' bilirubin. Direct bilirubin dissolves easily in water. Bilirubin which has passed through the liver is partly excreted into the gut in the bile salts which are needed in digestion. The brown colour of normal stools is partly due to bilirubin.

In jaundice either indirect or direct bilirubin, or both, may be increased. Jaundice is not a disease itself, but a sign caused by many disorders.

Causes of Jaundice

These may be divided into three major groups:-

a. Disorders causing an increase of indirect bilirubin: (often called pre-hepatic causes because they arise before the liver has been reached).

These are illnesses in which the red blood cells are broken down or haomolyscd, much more quickly than usual: so quickly in fact that although the liver is perfectly healthy, it cannot cope with the increase all at once.

The patient becomes jaundiced but his stools and urine will be of normal colour.

In newborn babies a common cause of this jaundice is 'rhesus haemolytic disease' in which the infants red blood cells are broken down because of a difference between his blood group and that of his mother.

In older infants and children the red blood cells may be an abnormal shape and this makes them more easily broken, e.g. they may be spherical as in congenital spherocytosis.

In both these examples because the red cells are broken down excessively, as well as becoming jaundiced the patient becomes anaemic. They often have very large livers and spleens.

The diagnosis of these diseases is made partly by finding a high indirect bilirubin in the blood stream and partly by finding abnormal red blood cells or incompatible blood groups in mother and child. Because indirect bilirubin dissolves readily in fat, if the level in the blood rises very high, bilirubin may deposit in the brain, which contains a lot of fat substances and may cause serious brain damage. This only happens with a *high* amount of *indirect* bilirubin and is not nowadays a common happening.

Treatment

In haemolytic disease of the newborn an 'exchange transfusion' is often required. In this the infant's blood, which contains the high indirect bilirubin, and the incompatible blood group factor, is gradually exchanged for blood which contains none of these, and which will also correct the anemia. The procedure may have to be repeated two or more times before the infants own blood stops being haemolysed: however, the condition will always improve and cure itself if the baby survives the initial days.

In disorders of red blood cell shape, blood transfusions are frequently needed. Sometimes the patient's spleen is removed because it appears to be in the spleen that most of the excessive breakdown of cells occurs. Taking out the spleen does not change their shape but it does prevent the anaemia and jaundice from being severe.

b. Disorders causing an increase of both indirect and direct bilirubin (often called hepatic causes because they arise when the liver itself is diseased).

If the liver cells are diseased then they cannot deal with even a normal amount of indirect bilirubin and so this builds up in the blood. When diseased, the cells often swell up and this blocks the passage into the gut of even that amount of bilirubin which has been converted to direct type: this direct bilirubin spills back into the blood stream and increases there too. Because less direct bilirubin reaches the gut the stools become pale: because there is an increase of direct bilirubin, which dissolves in water, in the blood, the excess comes out in the urine and so the urine appears dark brown.

The commonest cause of this type of jaundice in children is infective hepatitis.

This is due to a virus which is ingested by contaminations from a patient who suffered from the illness. The virus is excreted in the stools and urine of the patient for many weeks. The incubation period (from the time the virus gains entry to the time it causes obvious illness) is long—about thirty days.

The patient with infective hepatitis usually develops severe loss of appetite and may have pain in the liver area for several days before jaundice appears. His stools become pale, his urine dark and this persists until the jaundice days, or sometimes several weeks, later. Usually recovery is complete, but sometimes the liver is damaged permanently.

Treatment

There is no specific treatment. Bed rest is usually advised until the patient feels better. While they have no appetite the diet should be high in carbohydrate and low in fat (glucose fruit drinks are very satisfactory at this point).

c. Disorders causing an increase of direct bilirubin (often called post-hepatic or obstructive causes because they occur *after* the liver).

Bilirubin which the liver has converted from indirect to direct, is collected into channels called bile ducts and these pass it into the gall bladder where it is stored until passed into the gut.

Obstructive causes of jaundice are much commoner in old people than in paediatric practice but is seen occasionally as a distressing condition called *biliary atresia.* In this condition there are either no bile ducts or else they do not form together. All the direct bilirubin builds up therefore, and eventually spills back into the blood stream. The stools will obviously be very pale and the urine very dark.

Jaundice becomes evident soon after birth and deepens gradually and inevitably thence. Very rarely an operation may correct the bile duct deformity: usually the condition causes death in infancy.

Although jaundice is the most striking sign of liver disorder, the liver has many functions in addition to conversion of bilirubin and formation of bile salts. It has a role to play in metabolism and storage of protein, fat and carbohydrate: it also helps to break down certain drugs. However, illnesses which affect these functions are much less common than those resulting in jaundice.

31
Words to the Nurse

Whilst working in children's wards, the nurse must conduct herself with decorum. She should radiate tranquility and happiness while acting as the mother substitute at this time. It will not be necessary for her to shout in the wards, or to talk over a child's head, but to care for him thoughtfully and to include him in conservation, when caring for him. Kindness, a sympathetic ear, patience, a sense of humour, are amongst her essential qualities.

When the same nurse becomes the mother of her own child she will realise that her healthy thriving child is quite different from her sickly patients.

It is a difficult transition when you are mentally in tune with ill children.

The same kindness, patience and sympathy is required but the healthy child is a busy enquiring child seeking independence. The patient is glad to lean on 'his' nurse.

You will adjust to this, however,—as I have!—and each situation is richer for having had the other. It is just this reason that makes many mothers who come to nursing as a second career thoroughly sound members of the profession. As a ward sister I found this for myself.

A. M.

32
The Paediatric Nurse

A great deal of skill, patience, truthfulness, and understanding is required when nursing and caring for the sick child. The baby or very young child is unable to communicate with the nurse, so naturally this necessitates a keen sense of observation at all times.

On entering a children's ward for the first time the first impression may be one of noise and untidiness, but the nurse is usually aware of an atmosphere of happiness, even although there are ill patients in the ward.

When a child is admitted to the hospital, it is important to remember that this may be his first separation from his parents and family. He will be apprehensive whether he has been prepared for admission or not and he will need reassurance, combined with tender loving care.

The nurse should be quietly efficient when admitting the child as this allays the parents' fears as well as the patient's. He should always be called by his name, and if possible his mother may be allowed to help with the admission especially if he is difficult and crying. This helps separation to become a little easier.

Each procedure of the admission should be explained in detail to the child thus enabling him to orientate to his new surroundings. During admission the nurse can talk to him.

When he is tucked up in bed and all the particulars received from the parents they should be allowed to speak to their child. If he has a favourite toy or comforter these can be left with him. It is also advisable to find out from the parents any words that he may use for toilet requisites and also find out any food fads he may have.

It is quite natural for the child to cry on the departure of his parents, but invariably he will settle into the ward very quickly. If he is old enough the nurse can introduce him to the other children who are always pleased to make the new patient's acquaintance, and to share his toys!!!

Most children's hospitals have 'open' visiting hours. During these the parents can be encouraged to help by bathing, feeding and playing with their child—although they must be guided by the medical staff as to how much physical effort is allowable.

Other children are not usually allowed to visit paediatric wards due to the risk of them carrying infection into the ward. At present, this rule is being reviewed. The child should receive optimal care at all times. He should be helped with washing, cleaning teeth etc., and yet where he can do these things for himself he should be encouraged and supervised. Infected heads should be reported and treated.

All tests and procedures should be adequately explained. Older children are usually independent and enjoy helping the younger ones and the nursing staff. When possible or when the child's condition has improved sufficiently he is allowed up. This freedom is enjoyed. Discipline of over-active children is necessary. The nurse must realise that many of her patients come from very poor homes, where they have never been taught what is right or wrong. The child may have been spoiled due to repeated admissions to hospital. These are just two reasons for faulty behaviour.

Adequate sleep and rest is essential to aid recovery. The nurse will soon find out that most children sleep well and will not waken up during the busy bustle at night.

Babies will waken for feeds when they are hungry—night and day—and the nurse must remember that while he is in hospital she—the nurse—is the mother substitute and as such she requires to give him extra love, care and an occasional cuddle.

Ideally for the purpose of continuing the child's education while he is in hospital there should be a school room available to which the 'up' children can go for lessons. Children in bed who are well enough for school work will have lessons from the ward teacher.

Occupational therapy is also necessary—to keep the child interested and busy. Children can be encouraged to draw pictures, read books, write letters, and to use their hands making models etc. The nurse should always find time to take part in the children's games and play periods, although there are some ward helpers in some hospitals whose sole job is to be around to play with the children and share their games. However, she will be expected to know the Top Twenty, where the missing piece of the jigsaw puzzle is, and how to play various games.

The nurse can observe much of mental development from observing methods of play.

Toys should be in abundance in the ward. They should be robust and completely safe.

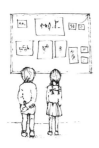

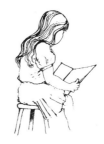

If there is a wall space in the ward a board may be erected. The children love drawing pictures to decorate it. They are proud when they see their efforts pinned up for all to see. An old clothes horse will be an excellent substitute.

Not every child is wanting to be swept up with communal activity so have a quiet little corner where a child can go with his book, jigsaw puzzle, colouring book—or even just to sit and watch the ward comings and goings.

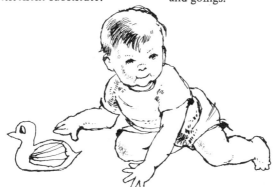

Younger children must play too. Mobile toddlers should have an equipped playroom supervised by a nursery nurse. Toys should be available to suit their age groups.

33
Reporting

It is of the utmost importance to read the reports relating to the progress of the children in the ward, and also to listen carefully to verbal reports given by sister or staff-nurse. When giving reports on handing over charge of the ward detailed accounts should be given.

When the nurse is in charge of the ward parents will ask her for information regarding their child's condition. It is essential that she gives an accurate and diplomatic account of the child's progress. Difficult parents or visitors will inevitably be encountered, and it is better to refer these parents to the person in charge, on return to duty. The nurse must always be sure to find out to whom she is speaking and not to assume that the persons visiting are the child's parents. No information should be given to anyone but the parents or official next of kin.

In medical wards the nurse should mark up the Kardex—or other record system—meticulously, i.e. refused feeds, types of vomiting, description of stools. Any change in the child's condition which is noted when working with him, should be reported.

ANSWERING THE TELEPHONE

When answering the telephone the nurse must first state the department in which she is working and then give her name. She should speak clearly and listen carefully. It is important that an exact message be taken to or from the person concerned.

When parents phone about their child, Sister should be told, and the information they get, given carefully and precisely. The patient's name should always be mentioned, and if advisable, and he is old enough he can be told when there have been inquiries for him. Calls from the police or the press should be referred to the administrative nursing staff or to the doctor.

34
The Dying Child

During her training the nurse will encounter acutely ill children and some of these children will inevitably die. This is very difficult to accept, and the nurse will find that no matter how often she is faced with death in a children's ward she will never become accustomed to it.

Naturally at this time the child will be given the optimum of care and his wishes granted within reason. Extra time should be spent with him and his family should be allowed to visit him at any time. Everything possible will be done to preserve his life, and drugs will be given to alleviate his pain.

The other children in the ward instinctively know when another child is very ill, and will speak to him and share their toys.

In the event of a death it is rare for them to ask questions but if they do it is advisable for the nurse to give a simple truthful answer if the child is old enough to understand, rather than to say that the child has gone home.

For obvious reasons some very ill or dying children will be nursed in side-wards or cubicles.

The parents too will require nurse's firm support and the nurse must be unobtrusive in her important role at this terminal stage. The parents must feel that they are very much included at this stage. Nurse must remember that in some cases she is probably very much younger than the parents or guardians and her mature competent handling of this trying stage in an illness will give those around her the maximum of moral support.

35
General Care of Children—Hygiene

Talking to Children

Each child should be treated as an individual, as they have their own personality. When talking to older children it is not necessary to speak 'baby language'. There is much more response if they are spoken to in an adult manner.

Before going off duty, children appreciate an individual 'good-night' from the nurse, with special reference to their own personal ailment, or praise can be given when they have responded especially well to some procedure or therapy. The same applies to 'good-morning'.

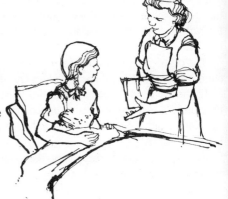

Toddlers always understand a smile and the nurse can speak to him with many reactions. Babies too, no matter how young, should be spoken to in a personal way. The nurse does not want to deprive the child emotionally of love and affection at this time especially.

Care of Nails

All children's nails should be kept short and clean. Nails are cut, when required to the shape of the fingers with blunt ended scissors. The nails when removed are placed on a swab. Dirt is removed with the blunt end of the scissors and wiped on a swab.

Babies nails are cut also when required as tiny infants may scratch themselves easily if nails are too long.

Bathing Children

Babies, toddlers and children are usually bathed every day. The procedure will be explained in the individual hospitals and will vary according to the condition of the child.

Care of Teeth

Teeth should be cleaned after every meal.

Each child, old enough to carry out this function by himself, or with help should have a toothmug, toothbrush and bowl kept behind his locker. His parents may provide toothpaste for him, but otherwise he can share from the hospital supply.

Occasionally a child will not know how to brush his teeth correctly. The following diagrams show the best way to train him.

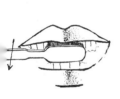 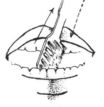 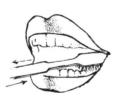

Brush from gum to tip—down for top teeth and up for lower teeth—i.e. one direction only (front).

Brush from gum to tip—down for top teeth and up for lower teeth—i.e. one direction only (back).

Brush along the tops of the back teeth—top and lower teeth.

Rinse out the mouth with clean water. Rinse out the toothbrush as well.

Care of Heads

Heads are usually inspected on admission to the ward, and then routinely at the ward Sister's discretion.

Requirements

A tray is set containing:-
1 Polythene sheeting cut to size
2 Bowl containing unsterile wool balls
3 Bowl for soiled wool balls containing appropriate disinfectant
4 Bowl for used combs also containing disinfectants
5 Suleo
6 Olive Oil
7 Combs (for routine inspection these may be kept behind the child's locker)
8 Fine-tooth combs

Method

The bed is screened and the procedure explained to the child. Polythene sheeting is tied round his shoulders. Ribbons or clasps are removed from girls if necessary. The hair is combed to remove tugs. With the fine-tooth comb in one hand, and cotton wool in the other, the hair is searched in sections commencing from the top of the head, combing down to the end. The toothcomb is turned up and wiped on to the swab and inspection takes place. The dirty wool is placed in the bowl containing disinfectant. Particular attention is paid to the nape of the neck, behind the ears, the crown of the head and to the hairline, as these are the commonest sites for lice and nits.

If the head is verminous or containing nits, appropriate lotion is applied as directed on the label of the bottle. The child's hair is then combed. The dirty comb is disinfected.

The clean head is also combed, and the comb is returned to the locker. All infected heads are reported.

Olive oil is applied to babies heads if there are scales on the scalp.

36
Feeding

Making up Feeds

In large children's hospitals feeds are usually made up in a milk kitchen and distributed at required intervals throughout the day. In smaller hospitals the nurses are responsible for making up of the feeds prior to feeding times. This procedure requires aseptic technique.

The nurse should wash her hands before preparing the feeds.

Each baby should have a Milton* bottle box in which is contained a bottle, a teat, and a polythene shield for the teat. These articles remain sterilised in the container between feeds. After inserting the articles completely in Milton solution it is four hours before they are completely sterilised. The very great advantage is also that mother can be trained to do this and continue it easily at home.

The other method of sterilisation may be employed, i.e. boiling.

The Milton method is a most reliable method of sterilisation.

Requirements

1 Boiled water from kettle (water should be at blood heat)
2 Plastic jug (previously sterilised). With mls. or oz. markings on the side
3 Whisk
4 Feeding Powder
5 Knife with which to level powder
6 Scoop
7 Sugar
8 Feeding instruction chart as prescribed by the physician

Method

The required amount of powder is measured in level scoops and put into the plastic jug. Sugar is added if ordered. A small amount of water

*Several other manufacturers produce equally effective sterilising agents which are also easily used in hospital or at home. Most manufacturers supply clear instructions.

is added and the mixture whisked to a smooth consistency. The correct amount of water is then added and mixed (usually scoop for scoop of water and powder is preferred). The feed is then transferred to the bottle, the teat applied by the neck, and the shield put on the teat to prevent contamination.

Feeding Ordinary Babies

1　The nurse should wash and dry her hands, after which she puts on the gown for the baby she is about to attend to. If necessary the infant is changed before. feeding. The napkin is put in a covered container if the baby is in a cubicle. The changing trolley is used if the baby is being nursed in an open ward; this should be put away before feeding begins.

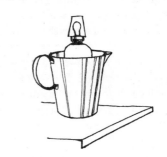

2　The nurse washes and dries her hands again.

3　The bottle containing the feed should be taken in a jug containing warm water to the baby's locker. A paper towel may be placed below this to prevent drips.

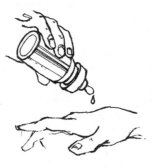

4　The temperature of the feed is tested by dropping a few drops of it on to the back of the nurse's hand. If the feed is too hot then it is cooled by allowing cold water to run over the bottle.

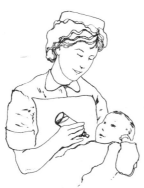

The baby is lifted from his cot. Both nurse and baby should be comfortably settled for the feed. Air should never enter the teat. Most babies enjoy a feed which is dropping at the rate of a drop per second from the teat. Sister will decide various sizes of holes required in difficult infants teats.

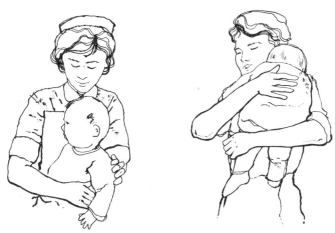

Several times during the feed the baby's wind should be broken. This is done by sitting the child on the knee while the nurse rubs between the shoulders, or leaning him on the nurse's shoulder with a rub from the waist up to the baby's shoulder. This takes several minutes and should *never* be hurried.

While winding the infant, the bottle should be placed in the jug and the teat shield placed on. When the baby is finished his feed, his wind is broken again. He is changed if required and his face should be washed. He can then be left comfortably in his cot. The baby will feel contented after his feed and will smile when spoken to.

The nurse must be relaxed when she is feeding the baby as if she is anxious she can transmit this to the infant which spoils the satisfaction of the feed.

5 The nurse again washes her hands. Drips are wiped from the locker top, and the bottle and teat are taken to the kitchen, where they are rinsed in cold water and cleaned with a bottle brush and hot soapy water. The articles are then replaced in *Milton (or sterilised as required in your hospital). It is important to make sure that the bottle is totally immersed to ensure adequate sterilisation. In larger hospitals the bottle is rinsed out, and sent back to the milk kitchen. The teat remains in the ward in separately labelled Milton (teat) containers.

6 The appropriate recordings are made in the Kardex, and if necessary a fluid intake and output chart is kept accurately. Any feeding difficulty is reported to Sister.

*See page 113.

eeding Difficult Babies

1 *Normal Babies*

If the baby has taken a substantial amount of mixed feeding before offering him the bottle the nurse may find that the infant will not finish his feed. The feed can then be offered to the baby 2-2½ hours later by which time he will probably be hungry. If he refuses the remainder completely the amount is recorded.

2 *Feeding Infants with Congenital Heart Disease*

Babies with congenital heart disease present many feeding problems for the nurse. These affected babies tire very easily, and usually have a poor sucking reflex. It is impossible to attempt feeding if the baby is agitated and breathless.

He should be made as comfortable as possible, and feeding is postponed until he is obviously hungry. It is essential that infants with cardiac abnormalities are given small amounts of milk frequently rather than large amounts at a time. The baby's colour should be observed during feeding as should signs of tiredness, dyspnoea, and distress. It is possible for the experienced nurse to help the baby suck by supporting his chin or cheek with her fingers.

When feeding becomes increasingly difficult the physician may order tube feeding. It is usually thought inadvisable to spoon feed because of the danger of weak babies inhaling the milk.

3 *Feeding Babies with Mongolism and Cretinism*

Due to the large size and protuberance of these infant's tongues feeding may prove difficult by bottle and teat. Due to mental deficiency in this instance the baby may be successfully tried with a cup and spoon.

4 Feeding Infants in Oxygen Tents and Croupettes

If the infant becomes very distressed outside his oxygen or humidity supply the tent should be kept as near closed as possible during feeding to preserve its oxygen or humidity content. While feeding inside the tent he should be propped up against the pillows and his head supported by the nurse.

In very distressed babies, tube feeding may be indicated. Careful observation is required.

5 Feeding Babies in Incubators

The baby remains in the incubator while he is being fed. The tray that he is being nursed on may be tilted to the required angle for him. The nurse gains access to the child by opening the ports at the front of the incubator. The baby's head is supported by the nurse's hand, and the bottle manoevred with the other.

6 Feeding Babies with Hiatus Hernia

A baby with this condition is usually nursed in a 'baby-sitter' box, in an endeavour to prevent vomiting occurring so frequently. Thirty minutes before feeding he is given an antacid drug to neutralise the hydrochloric acid in the stomach. He is then fed in the normal way with a thickened feed and returned upright—after breaking his wind—to the box.

7 Babies who Ruminate

Babies who ruminate (i.e., the infant receives pleasure by voluntarily regurgitating into his mouth part of his feed, which he chews and sometimes vomits) may also be nursed in these boxes. Plastic shields can be used for their hands to prevent them putting their fingers into their mouths. The feeding regime of these babies is the same as for babies with hiatus hernia.

Tube Feeding

There are several ways of feeding by tube. The method used depends on the reason for giving artificial feeds, e.g.

a. Prematurity

b. Respiratory distress causing inability to suck normally

c. Congenital heart defects with congestive cardiac failure causing breathlessness, exhaustion, and cyanosis with subsquent feeding difficulty

This method of feeding may be performed at regular intervals by passing a tube through one nostril to the lower end of the oesophagus.

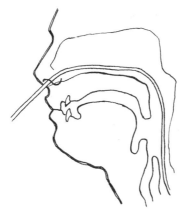

The tube is removed when the feed is finished.

This is a fairly skilled procedure and the pupil nurse will not often be asked to perform it. However, it is wise to know the commoner reasons for it to be employed.

Medicines

Medicine should never be added to feeds. As the child may not completely finish its feed.

37

Administration of Oral Medicines

A great deal of attention and concentration is required when administering medicines. Nowadays, however, this task is made much easier as there are many drugs made in a more palatable form suitable for use in the paediatric wards.

1 The nurse should stay with the patient until she is satisfied that the entire dose of drug is swallowed.

2 The medicine trolley should not be left unattended in the ward.

3 Drugs should never be given to children unless written up by the physician.

Older Children

After explaining the reason why the drug is being given the nurse will find that most children are invariably willing to take their pills or mixture without fuss. Tablets can be crushed and put on top of Rose Hip Syrup to make it easier for the child to swallow. A drink or a sweet if allowed can be given after medicine to remove the taste. Praise is given to the child for his co-operation.

Toddlers

Patience is required with younger children especially when the child is having medicine for the first time. The nurse puts his feeder on and while doing so should talk to him, smile and encourage him.

When toddlers are used to taking medicine they usually do so quite well, and look forward to a drink or sweet afterwards!!!

✷ Babies

Babies can be difficult. The nurse should pour out the medicine first. She should put on the gown used for working with the particular baby, and ties on his feeder. He should be picked up if possible and wrapped in a blanket to keep his hands out of reach. It is more convenient to give an infant the drug in small quantities on a spoon which should be held near the mouth to catch any spills. His face should be wiped afterwards and a drink can also be given.

Medicine Rounds

This is part of the routine of the day and is done at regular intervals—Nurse must note that sometimes it is necessary to deal in a special way with individual drugs.

Administration of Special Drugs

Some drugs are administered at special times without medicine rounds in order that they may be maximally effective. The more common ones in this category are mentioned below:-

Digoxin

It is a rule in most hospitals that the apex beat is taken before giving digoxin to children with cardiac failure. The beat is recorded by listening through a stethoscope to the heart beat for *one full minute* when the child is at rest. The fourth intercostal space at the nipple line is where the apex beat is found. Slowing of the apex beat may show that the child is suffering from digoxin overdose—but this slowing may be due to other causes as well.

Abnormalities of the beat would be reported to the ward sister who, in turn would notify the medical staff.

Aluminium Hydroxide Gel

This drug is used in the treatment of peptic ulcer or hiatus hernia and is known as an alkali or antacid. It can be given to the patient either before, after, or with meals to neutralise the hydrochloric acid in the stomach thus treating one of the main factors in causing the ulcer.

Pancrex V Powders or Capsules

This drug is given to children suffering from fibrocystic disease of the pancreas. It is oral pancreatin which replaces the pancreatic enzymes. Both types may be sprinkled over food—(the capsule form being separated). They can also be made more palatable by mixing the powder with Rose Hip Syrup or water and then given to the child half an hour before meals. If the powder is on the food then the nurse should feed or stay with the child until he has eaten the food containing the pancrex powder. Children with this condition soon become used to the taste of this drug and take it without trouble. The powders should be stored in well-closed containers as, if left in a damp atmosphere, they are likely to become lumpy when Rose Hip Syrup or water is added.

Several drugs are now quoted which warrant mention because of their method of administration.

Isoprenaline

This drug is used in the treatment of bronchial spasm in asthmatic patients and given sub-lingually so that it is absorbed slowly and steadily into the blood stream. An explanation should have been given to the child before giving the drug.

Aspirin

Aspirin—when given to a child should be given with a glass of milk as this aids its absorption and also prevents gastric erosion. It is for this reason that aspirin should either be crushed or halved. Watch that a quantity of the drug is not lost when it is being crushed.

Sulphonamides

Copious fluids should be given to children who are having these drugs.

Large doses of Sulphonamides may become concentrated in the kidney and this will result in solid crystals forming. The crystals block the renal tubules causing haematuria and anuria.

Steroids

Prednisolone, cortisone acetate, corticotrophin (A.C.T.H.) etc., come under this group. They control the processes of allergy and inflammation and are beneficial when treating numerous conditions. It is unfortunate that prolonged usage produces side-effects. Therefore, observation must be made for:-

1. Oedema caused by salt retention.
2. Daily urine testing should be carried out for 'sugar' as diabetes mellitus may be precipitated.
3. Cushingism with 'moonface' buffalo pad, acne, hirsutism.
4. If the drug is withdrawn suddenly adrenal collapse would result, due to the natural secretion of cortisone becoming diminished, as the adrenal gland becomes inert.

38
Giving Injections

It is important that a truthful explanation is given to the young patient regarding injections as usually a child has great fear of this procedure.

The nurse should explain that the injection will hurt a little, but that it will not take long to give. In medical wards children frequently receive several injections on admission as an aid to diagnosis, and the nurse should always be there to comfort them at this time.

It is preferable that the preparations for giving injections should be carried out in a treatment room, as the sight of syringes and needles are frightening to the child who is about to receive the injection, and to the other children in the ward.

Aseptic precautions are taken.

When the child is having injections as treatment two nurses should always be present—one who will give it, and the other who will hold, prepare, and reassure the patient.

Most children will cry when the needle is inserted, or when the drug is injected. At this time he should be consoled and extra praise and affection given.

Older childer can be very brave at this time.

Injection Sites

 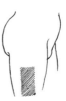

1. The lateral aspect of the thigh, or upper outer quadrant of the buttock is used when administering intra-muscular injections.
2. The deltoid muscle is usually used when giving hypodermic injections, but in diabetic patients the site is varied because the injections are given so frequently.

   If the same site was used, pain, bruising, and oedema would result.

39
Recording of Temperature Pulse and Respiration Rates (T.P.R.)

Temperatures

In children's medical wards temperatures are usually taken rectally with a clinical thermometer which has a short thick bulb. This is the safest type of thermometer to use when taking rectal temperature readings, as it is less liable to break. The normal rectal temperature is 99°F or 37°C.

Requirements

1. Each individual child should have a thermometer for his exclusive use. These can be kept disinfected in a named glass test tube on a thermometer tray. This tray should contain gallipots for clean and soiled swabs.
2. In his locker the child should have a K.Y. jelly lubricant pack.
3. The changing trolley is required.
4. The Kardex or record card should be available into which the recordings are entered.

Method

An explanation must be given to the child as he will be afraid that this procedure will cause pain. He should be asked to lie in the left lateral position, after which he is covered with a blanket to prevent perplexity and embarrassment

The infant's temperature can be recorded efficiently if he is lain on his back with his legs raised vertically. The thermometer is wiped dry with a clean swab and shaken down to below 35°C (95°F).

The bulb is then moistened with lubricating jelly and inserted into the rectum—one inch for infants and one and a half inches for older children. The thermometer should be held firmly and the buttocks squeezed together for the time required to register the mercury. The thermometer is then wiped clean, and read. The mercury is shaken down, the thermometer is then returned to its compartment on the tray. The nurse washes and dries her hands before recording in the Kardex, and going on to the next patient.

Normal Pulses and Respiration Rates

The average readings for these rates will be seen on page 10.

Pulses

It is important to take the child's pulse when he is in bed or sitting on a chair, as hyperactivity or crying results in inaccuracy. The nurse should feel for the radial pulse with her first two fingers. The pulse is counted for one full minute observing the rhythm, rate and quality of the beat. It is difficult to record a toddler's pulse if he is younger than two years of age, unless he is asleep. It can be felt at the temple. A pulse beat may be noticeable at the anterior fontanelle in babies.

Sleeping Pulses

This is the most accurate way of recording the pulse rate. It is particularly helpful in estimating the progress of children who suffer from rheumatic fever. Again the pulse rate should be counted for one full minute. The child should be disturbed as little as possible. The sleeping pulse is taken routinely every night and usually recorded with a ring round it in the Kardex.

Respiration Rates

Respirations cannot be counted if the child is crying. It is advisable to total the respirations of older children immediately after recording the pulse rate. Sometimes they are aware that the nurse is counting the respiration rate, and this may produce unnatural respiratory rates.

Children suffering from acute chest conditions should have their pyjama jacket removed in order that careful observation of the type of inspiration and expiration made as this is an important feature for observation.

Bowel Movement

This information is usually gathered at T.P.R. time. Older and mobile children can be asked if their bowels have moved as it is virtually impossible for the nurse to observe this function each time when the child is an 'up' patient in the ward.

Potty Training

It will be remembered that the nurse has ascertained from parents if there is any special word that the child uses when he needs to be potted. Due to concern and fear of all that is unknown and strange, young children who have been toilet-trained at home sometimes regress when they come into hospital. In this instance they should never be rebuked when they are wet or soiled, but offered a potty at regular intervals throughout the day. Ideally one nurse may be allocated to this function, thus letting the child feel secure with the person doing this for him but failing this at each changing round the nurses can pot the toddlers on the way round the ward.

If their stay in hospital is to be short, children who have not been toilet-trained before their admission to hospital should not have potty training attempted while they are there, as this will just frighten and confuse them, and any efforts would prove unsuccessful. However, it is frequently found that with the regular potting at reasonable times in the ward that some children who are hospitalised for a long time, may achieve a toilet routine. This deserves praise and a lot of encouragement.

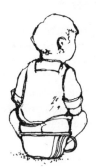

Changing of Babies and Toddlers

Usually there are routine times for changing rounds in most wards but naturally when a child needs changing it is done as soon as possible.

Requirements

Changing trolley containing:-

1. linen, napkins, powder, cream, disinfectant, enco-wipes, bag for soiled napkins and linen.
2. Buggy for linen.

Method

The changing trolley—or equivalent— is taken to the bedside. The wet or soiled napkin is removed and put into the bag provided.

The infant's towel is placed below his buttocks. Faeces, stale talcum powder and cream are removed using enco-wipes which have been soaked in warm soapy water. The nurse can wash the buttocks and genitalia with her hand. Observation is made for dermatitis, broken areas, or excoriation. This is reported. The appropriate remedy will be prescribed and applied.

Careful drying takes place making sure that all crevices are dry. Talcum alone is applied if the buttocks are in good condition. The napkin is then put on around the buttocks,—the pin fastened horizontally.

Vomiting

Changing after Vomiting

Nurse must remember to take water to wash the patient when she takes a clean napkin and linen to the bedside and a bucket for the soiled articles. If the child has vomited he should be thoroughly washed, dried and powdered, in the appropriate areas before putting on his clean linen.

Make sure also that his nose is clean as frequently when a child is being sick vomit will flow down the nose as well as be projected from the mouth.

It is also refreshing for the child to have a mouth wash following a vomiting episode.

The child who has been vomiting needs to be reassured and once he is cleaned and tidied again he should be settled and left to rest.

Before disposing of the child's vomit it is wise to enquire whether or not an observation specimen of it is required.

40
Prevention of Accidents

Care must be taken at all times to prevent accidents as children are particularly prone and vulnerable. A few of the more commonly found hazards are mentioned below:-

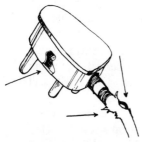

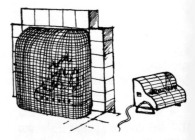

1 Flexes should be in excellent condition on all electrical apparatus. Requisition must be made at once to the electrician to repair faulty plugs, sockets, flexes and switches.

2 Open fires (where they are still in use), or electric fires in wards should be safely guarded using one of the well tried and officially accepted fire preventions societie fire guards.

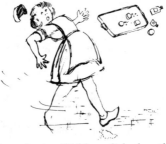

3 Floors should not be too highly polished so that accidents involving slipping and falling can be avoided. Any water, juice or other spill should be wiped up immediately as some of these liquids are every bit as dangerous on the floor surface as a highly glazed polish.

4   Window cords and blind cords should hang will out of reach.

5   Cotsides should never be left down even for a moment, if the child is unattended, as active infants could fall out quickly and easily. The sides should be replaced and locked immediately after working with the child.

6   Medicines and drugs should always be kept under lock and key out of reach. So many capsules and tablets are manufactured in attractive shapes, colours, and sizes that they are naturally attractive to the child.

7   If gifts are brought to the children wrapped in polythene bags these should be removed immediately.

8   Hot water bottles should be filled with water under boiling point. The bottles should not be filled too full. Make sure they are securely fastened. It is wise to put a cover on the bottle.

9   When preparing the bath for children some <u>cold water</u> is run into the bath first. The temperature of the water should be checked carefully by the nurse, and by the child if he is old enough.

10 Patients should not be allowed into the kitchen unless accompanied by a nurse or orderly.

11 Low windows should have guard rails or protection of some kind in front of them and others should open from the top.

12 If there are plants or flowers on the window ledge, make sure that they are out of reach of the children.

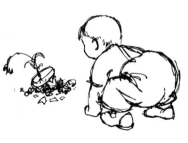

41

Weighing and Measuring of Children

In medical wards particularly recording of children's height and weight is extremely important. The doctor can estimate the child's condition and progress from these recordings which may also help in the diagnosis of various diseases.

Weighing Babies

If possible on admission both height and weight are recorded. Metric scales are in use in most hospitals. Children should be weighed undressed.

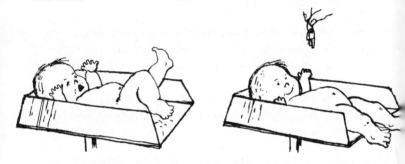

When weighing crying or struggling babies it is necessary to distract him with a noisy object. This is necessary as an acurate weight can only be recorded when the infant is almost motionless.

All children are weighed once per week but some patients' diagnosis requires weighing twice weekly.

Babies and very young children are usually weighed every day.

Measuring Babies

Two nurses are required when a baby's height is being measured using the centimetre stick. To obtain a truly accurate reading the baby must be as immobile as possible. The height is measured on a flat surface and the child lies on his back.

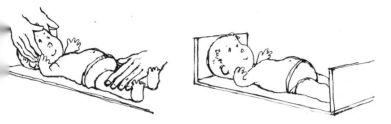

One nurse holds his head in contact with a board at the head of the
ick while the other nurse holds his legs straight with the feet at right
ngles to the legs. She then brings the sliding board up against the baby's
eels.

Weighing and Measuring Children

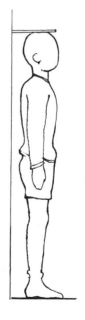

Scales for older children have a
measuring stick attached at right angles
to the base plate which makes recording
eight relatively simple. The height should
be recorded by asking the child to stand
with his heels in contact with the back of
he scales. He should have his shoes off
nd his head is positioned so that he looks
straight forward. The sliding stick is moved
own to touch the top of the child's head.
He is asked to stand as tall as possible,
with arms at his side.

In some hospitals, children are measured
n a special table which is easier when the
child is unable to stand. Long term
patients should be measured once monthly.
Any discrepancy found when carrying out
outine weighing and measuring should be
hecked by a senior nurse.

42
Collection of Urine Specimens

Urine specimens are required frequently in medical wards as the results can give valid information regarding diagnosis, e.g. in urinary infections, nephritis, diabetes mellitus, Henoch Schonlein purpura, phenylketonuria.

Collection of Single Urine Specimens from Infant Boys and Girls

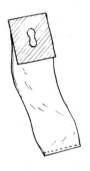 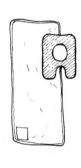

Requirements
1 Disposable chiron or 'U' bag. The latter being the most reliable as there will be no back flow of urine if the baby is active.
2 Changing trolley.
3 Scissors.
4 Labelled urine glass.

Method
1 The baby's napkin area is washed, and thoroughly dried to make sure that the urine bag will adhere.
2 The protective backing from the adhesive is removed.
3 The sides of the urine bag are separated.
4 The adhesive side is pressed around the external genitalia.

Care should be taken with boys to ensure that the penis is well inserted into the hole provided, and that it is not too tight. The adhesive should not stick to the scrotum.

In girls the hole should be placed adequately over the vulva area.

The clean napkin is then pinned on. To collect the specimen the bag is taken off carefully. Any traces of adhesive are removed with a swab soaked in methylated ether.

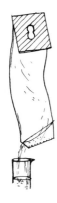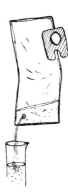

The corner of the Chiron bag is cut off and the urine allowed to run into a urine glass. With a 'U' bag the appropriate blue square is torn off and the urine flows into the glass.

All urine glasses should be labelled and then taken to the test room. The doctor should be notified that the specimen has been obtained, as he will want to test it while it is fresh.

Cleaned-up Specimens

If a sterile specimen of urine is required from infants for bacteriological purposes extra sterile equipment is needed to clean the external genitalia.

1　Gallipot containing sterile saline.
2　Gallipot for wool balls.
3　Bowl for used swabs.
4　Remainder of requisites as for previous specimen.

Preparing Boys

First the nurse washes and dries her own hands. The penis should be gently washed with sterile saline and swabs, pulling back the foreskin in order that it is cleaned. It is then dried prior to carrying out the collection routine as described on page 133.

Preparing Girls

Initially the nurse washes and dries her hands. The vulva is cleaned using a separate swab for each part and for drying. The nurse guides the swab from above downwards to prevent infection spreading from the vagina to the perineum and also to the urethra. The bag is applied as before. When urine is passed it is transferred to a sterile labelled bacteriological urine container, and despatched to the laboratory with the appropriate request form.

Mid-Stream Specimen of Urine

Mid-stream specimens of urine are obtained from older children. The 'mid-stream' of urine is regarded as the part least likely to contain bacteria. An explanation is given to the child and he is reassured that the procedure is very simple and will not hurt at all.

Boys

Requirements as for 'cleaned-up-specimens' from male infants, with the addition of a bed bottle and a sterile foil bowl. The genitalia are cleaned as before. The child is asked to micturate into the bottle, and then to stop. The middle stream of the urine is then collected into the bowl. The child then completes voiding into the urinal.

If the boy is up and about, then this procedure can be performed successfully in the toilet.

The urine is then sent in its labelled sterile bottle to the laboratory with suitable request form.

Girls

Requirements as for 'cleaned-up-specimens' from female infants plus a bedpan and a sterile foil tray. The bed is screened. The external genitalia cleaned as before. The child is asked to pass urine into the bedpan, stop, the middle of the urine is passed into the foil tray and the end of the flow voided into bedpan. The specimen is then bottled, labelled, and sent to the laboratory as before.

Twenty-Four Hour Collection of Urine

These are required for further investigation into certain conditions, e.g. rickets, phenylketonuria, adrenal hyperplasia. Collection of urine for twenty-four hours from the older child is simple if explicit directions have been given to him. His urine is collected in a urinal each time he micturates and put into the appropriate winchester jar sent from Biochemistry. This usually contains preservative. A SAVE ALL URINE sign should be fixed to the bed.

To collect large amounts of urine from toddlers and babies Chiron or 'U' bags are used. The method of application is described on page 133. The upper part of the bag may have a split made in it in order that a catheter may be inserted, into the bag. The urine can then be aspirated, with a 20 ml. syringe, and put in a foil bowl from which it is poured into the winchester. This prevents the bag having to be changed each time that urine is passed with resultant preservation of the skin area.

Ideally one nurse should be responsible for the urine collection. She should attend to the child frequently to make sure that he is comfortable and to see that all urine is saved.

If small amounts are lost the approximate amount is recorded, and the biochemist informed by the ward sister so that this may be taken into account during the accurate assessment of the specimen. If large amounts of urine are lost the collection will have to be abandoned.

On completion of the collection the winchester plus the biochemistry request form is sent to the laboratory.

43
Collection of Stools

Stools are collected for several reasons in the medical wards, e.g. estimation of fat output, faecal occult blood, stool acidity test, tryptic activity and examination for parasites. These findings are an important aid to diagnosis in certain illnesses.

SAVE ALL STOOLS

A SAVE ALL STOOLS sign should be displayed prominently on the bed of the child involved. If the test can be performed in the ward the soiled napkin is placed in a covered container and left in the test room.

For biochemical tests a square of polythene cut to the size of the napkin can be inserted when the napkin is put on the child. This makes

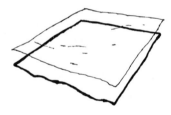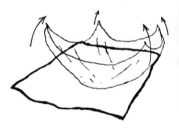

it a simple task to put the stool and the polythene into a faeces container before sending it to the laboratory for analysis.

Prolonged stool collections using polythene, usually leaves the buttocks red, which may be treated after completion of the test.

Hygiene during taking of Specimens

It cannot be stressed too often that nurse must be scrupulously reful about the washing of her hands during the taking of specimens. he should also insist that her young patient follows her example he is old enough. If he is not then she must see that it is done or him.

44
Serving of Meals

Meals for sick children should be served attractively and in small quantities. The child will ask for more, and the toddler will cry if he is still hungry.

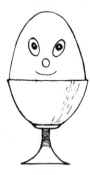

Why not draw a funny face on a boiled egg?

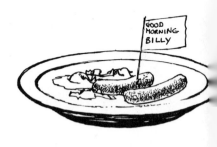

A personal notice on a stick stuck in a sausage!!!

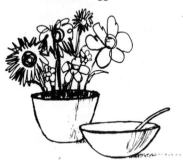

A small dish of flowers will charm a little girl.

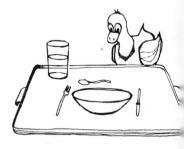

Sit a favourite toy on the tray to watch child eating.

At each main meal milk should be given to drink to children who are not on a special diet.

Children should never be forced to drink or eat—but encouraged as much as possible. The child who is particularly reluctant to eat may benefit from being given food that he especially likes which can be obtained on request from the kitchen. Diet permitting, older children can be given a choice of the foods available.

Pelican Bib

Toddlers should wear feeders. A particularly good shape of feeder is as illustrated alongside.

Made in pliable plastic with a deep open pocket at its base, to catch the dropped food!!!

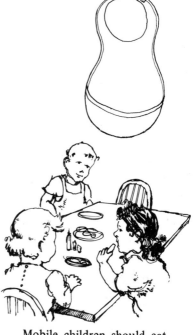

Feeding Toddlers

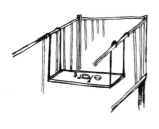

When toddlers are being fed in bed they should have a table erected over the cot sides. These should not be put up until immediately before the meal is served to prevent accidents.

Mobile children should eat around the table. This adds a pleasant interlude to life in the ward and frequently children—who on their own in bed—seemed to have little zest for eating—eat much better when they have company.

Children in bed may eat from bed tables.

Spoon Feeding

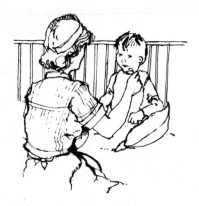

The nurse should sit when spoon feeding as it is psychologically upsetting for the child if she stands. It creates a feeling of rush and impatience which is upsetting. He can be placed on the nurse's knee or he may be fed while sitting in his cot. Care should be taken that food is cool when given to younger children. Toddlers like soft foods. The addition of gravy to main courses is usually popular.

Children Helping

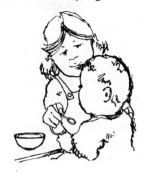

Provided the little convalescent child has had her own complete meal she might then help feed some of her smaller ward-mates.

In most medical wards, following lunch, the curtains or blinds are closed and the children rest for an hour.

Balanced Diet

It is important that patients receive a well balanced diet, containing the essential food requirements for recovery.

1 Loss of Appetite

It must also be remembered that when a child is ill he will probably have lost his appetite, and during the initial stages of his illness he may only want to drink a lot of fluid.

2 Visitors and Food

It is a rule in most children's hospitals that parents and visitors should hand in gifts of sweets, food and fruit to the ward sister, who will see that these are distributed properly at appropriate times. Visitors are not usually permitted to feed the patients between meals.

Special Diets

```
SPECIAL  DIET
```

A 'SPECIAL DIET' notice should be fixed to the bed as a constant reminder to the staff and visitors that the child must not receive ordinary food.

In large hospitals the staff in the Diet Kitchen deal with the preparation and calculation of special diets, while in smaller hospitals the ward sister herself may be responsible for this preparation. Direction in this case will be given to sister by the physician in charge.

To treat children with special diets the nurse must be aware of the reasons for giving and omitting certain foods. Many older children too can be told very simply why they may not eat certain things.

Diet Sheets

There are diet sheets available in hospitals to which she can refer. The parents can be instructed as to which brands of sweets and drinks to bring for their child.

Home Follow-Up

Parents must receive sufficient instructions from the dietician to ensure complete understanding before dismissal of their child from hospital.

Supervision of the child is maintained at the outpatient clinic.

15
Special Diets

Some of the more common diets are mentioned briefly:-

Gluten-Free Diet in Coeliac Disease

As the child cannot absorb the gluten which is found in wheat flour, this substance should be completely excluded from the diet. The main forbidden foods in this group are—bread, cakes, biscuits, sausages, semolina and certain sweets.

Bread, cakes and biscuits which are baked using gluten free flour can be given at liberty.

The diet is fairly unrestricted as there are many foods which can be given and eaten freely. There is also a wide variety of gluten free foods produced in proprietary forms available.

These children receive vitamin supplements also.

2 Diabetic Diet in Diabetes Mellitus

In diabetic patients the mechanism of insulin production is impaired. This means that the child needs to have injections of individually calculated doses of insulin daily.

The diet must not be allowed to vary in its constituents. Meals must be taken at regular intervals as postponement of food may result in hypoglycaemia.

A suitable snack in consultation with the ward sister can be allowed between meals but sweets, cakes, sugar and chocolates are forbidden.

Nowadays there are several varieties of 'diabetic' drinks and sweets may be given instead of those containing sugar.

Each diabetic child's diet is different depending on his individual requirements. Measured amounts of carbohydrate according to the child's weight is often prescribed. The total amount may be divided into 10. gm. portions which makes interchange of carbohydrate foods easy for the parents.

Although restriction of carbohydrate is the main factor in the diet, it is very important that the child receives protein, fat, fruit, and average helpings of vegetables containing little or no carbohydrate.

3 Bland Diet in Peptic Ulcer

It is sometimes thought that the diet given to help treat patients with peptic ulcers is ineffective. Most children, however, do experience alleviation from pain on a bland diet.

This should contain non-irritating foods. Milk is given with and between meals. Foods to avoid are those which are highly spiced, indigestable, greasy or fatty. Coarse vegetables, pips and skins of fruit, sauces and condiments should also be evaded.

Extra vitamin C is given in the form of oranges, and orange drinks as the diet as outlined is lacking in this.

It is important to see that small meals are given frequently rather than large meals at spaced out intervals.

4 Restricted Fluids, Sodium, and Protein Diet in Acute Nephritis

An important function of the kidneys is to excrete protein in waste product form. In acute nephritis protein is restricted to rest the kidneys

Also in order to rest the diseased kidneys restricted fluids are given initially. Half strength milk (30-40 fluid ounces or 900-1,200 millilitres) is offered to the child daily. A detailed fluid intake and output chart is maintained.

Boiled sweets may be given freely to ensure an adequate calorie intake.

When diuresis occurs and there is a reduction in haematuria, a cereal diet is begun. This consists of cereals, potatoes, fruit, vegetables, puddings, bread, butter, and jam.

As the patient recovers and the urine clears, light diet is given— including protein. Normal diet is substituted in the convalescent stages.

5 Low Salt, restricted Fluids, and High Protein Diet in Nephrosis

At the commencement of treatment fluids are reduced to 30-40 fluid ounces (900-1,200 millilitres) daily as at this stage the child will be oedematous. For this reason also the sodium is restricted to less than 2 grams per day. An increased amount of protein is given to help to balance the albuminuria.

When the symptoms have disappeared then the restrictions are gradually removed on medical instruction.

6 Low Phenylalanine Diet in Phenylketonuria

In this condition the liver lacks an enzyme which helps the body to use phenylalanine (a normal part of protein).

Because the enzyme is not effective phenylalanine builds up in the bloodstream and has poisonous effects—especially on the brain.

Dietary treatment aims to limit the amount of phenylalanine (protei (protein) ingested. The daily maximum is very small compared with ordinary diet as phenylalanine is a part of all natural protein.

Artificially prepared protein foods have to be used and the method of preparation means that vitamins must be given.

The diet is expensive and complicated. Artificial foods are commonly used. For babies food is prepared in liquid form. It will not, however, support normal health or growth without added phenylalanine ordered by the physician as measured milk.

For older children it is prepared as puddings flavoured with fruit crushes, or soups flavoured with tomato juice.

The diet is restricted as it consists mainly of fruit and vegetables. The few foods which are phenylalanine free may be given as lib, e.g. low P.A. bread and biscuits, tea, coffee, syrup, jam, marmalade, sno snowcrest jelly, lemon and orange squash, rose hip syrup etc.

An accurate account of refusals and replacements of protein-containing foods given would be kept.

46
Intravenous Fluids

Nursing of Children with Intravenous Infusions

Intravenous fluids are either given into a vein by venepuncture, or into a vein which has been incised with a scalpel. This second method is usually employed when some degree of difficulty has been encountered with the first method.

This procedure is performed by a doctor.

Reasons for Administering Intravenous Fluids

1 To correct dehydration and electrolyte imbalance, as the child is usually vomiting and is therefore unable to tolerate oral fluids.
2 To replace blood loss, e.g., in leukaemia, aplastic anaemia, injury.

Management of Intravenous Infusion

Younger or agitated ill children will probably require sedation. Older patients co-operate willingly if a suitable explanation and reassurance is given.

The sleeve or pyjama trousers are removed before beginning, depending on which vein is selected. The child is observed carefully during the procedure.

On completion he should be kept warm and frequent checks should be made that the method of limb immobilisation is not too tight. It may be necessary to errect a bed cradle over the limb to minimise the weight of the bedclothes from the site.

An accurate intake and output chart is kept (see page 155) and an hourly check of the fluid running in intravenously is recorded. The physician will decide how much fluid the child needs and he will also indicate the rate of flow.

The level of the infusion bottle—wnen the older type of apparatus is used—is watched carefully as the bottle should never be allowed to empty completely—this prevents air entry to the circulation.

It is somewhat easier to regulate the Metriset which is used more commonly in intravenous infusion in infants, e.g. The advantage of this type of set is that it may be adjusted so that the number of drops delivered per minute equals the number of mls. infused per hour, e.g. fifteen drops per minute gives fifteen mls. per hour, i.e. the infusion enters at a constant rate throughout the prescribed time.

Two nurses must check the label on the new bottle of fluid before setting it up. The tube is clamped prior to the change. A state Registered nurse must supervise the changing of the intravenous blood or its derivatives. The child should receive extra special care and understanding at this time and a diligent watch is made by the nurse for any abnormality or complication which may arise, e.g.

1 Swelling.
2 Spasm of vein causing slowing of rate of flow.

Observation of Patient having Intravenous Blood

Nurse should watch for any of the following complications:-

1 Swelling.

2 Spasm of vein causing slow rate of flow.

3 Elevation of temperature.

4 Rash.

5 Respiratory distress.

6 Shivering in excess.

7 Convulsions.

47
Oxygen Therapy

Nursing Children in Croupettes

Children are nursed in a croupette when they are suffering from severe respiratory distress.

Respirations in—bronchitis, bronchiolitis, laryngeal stridor, croup, etc., are improved. The tent can be used with oxygen, humidity, and or air depending on the condition to be treated. A diapump may be used in conjunction with the croupette, into which compressed filtered air is blown forcibly, through distilled water to form a fine spray or vapour. The tent should be assembled according to the manufacturer's instruction, which will accompany the croupette. Care should be taken that a large pile of pillows do not block the portal entry of air. The canopy should be tucked in adequately to make certain that the correct requirements of oxygen or humidity concentration are received.

The humidity jar should be watched frequently to ensure that a sufficient level of water is maintained.

In specialised cases the doctor may order alternative solutions as treatment. If the child is febrile, ice and cold water can be poured into the trough to establish a moderately cold temperature.

To prevent overflowing the end of the outlet tube should be attached to the trough and drained as the ice melts.

A thermometer is inserted into the tent. This registers temperature.

An adequate explanation of the procedure and a great deal of reassurance is given to the older child to minimise his fears. Children of all ages should never be left unattended until they have become quite used to these surroundings. If the child is in any way afraid or upset, it would of course result in respiratory distress, and this would defeat the whole purpose of the treatment. Careful observation is required and the nurse should always be near to attend to the child's needs. Soft toys and books may be played with. His clothing and linen should be changed at regular intervals, as there is a tendency to frequent dampness from condensation.

The ports or zips at the side of the tent are opened to gain easy access to the patient. He remains in the croupette until signs of respiratory distress are minimal. He receives visitors as usual.

Nursing Children in Oxygen Tents

Inhalation of oxygen is essential to life. Deficiencies of oxygen can occur in, e.g. congenital heart disease with congestive heart failure, respiratory obstruction, disease of the lung, and certain types of poisoning. This deficiency is counteracted by the use of oxygen therapy.

Methods of Administering Oxygen—Babies in Incubators.

Babies in incubators can receive oxygen therapy from the pipeline supply which is metered by the incubator flow meter from where it passes to the oxygen jet assembly.

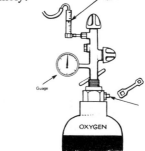

The oxygen flow rates should be read from the incubator flow meter only, and not the pipeline flow meter.

A reliable oxygen concentration analyser is used. No infant or child should receive oxygen in a greater concentration than he needs, or for longer than is needed.

Oxygen therapy is ordered by the physician.

Methods of Administering Oxygen—Babies in Cots or Children in Beds.

Oxygen tents are used for babies in cots or older children in bed. The canopy is placed over the bed or cot and tucked in properly all round. A receptacle for ice is hung at the back of the bed. The ice keeps the atmosphere in the tent cool. The ice will melt into the lower compartment, the water must be emptied as necessary.

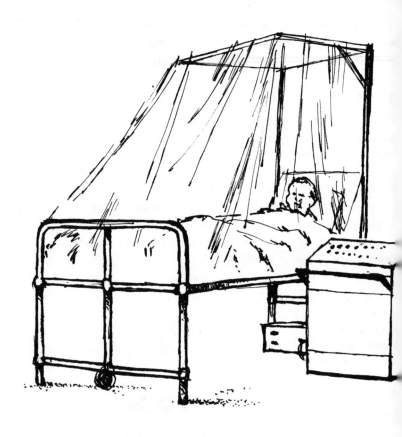

To gain access to the patient the nurse uses the pockets at either side of the tent. The oxygen concentration and the temperature of the tent are checked as before.

The child should be reassured that he is safe in the tent so that he will gain confidence and become unafraid.

He can play with toys which are non-mechanical as mechanical types will cause sparkes, which of course in the circumstances is a fire hazard.

Strict fire precautions must be adhered to as combustion will occur without difficulty in the presence of oxygen.

48
Infectious Diseases

Children who develop infectious fevers, e.g., measles, chicken pox, rubella, etc., are transferred to an infectious disease Hospital, where they are nursed until free from infection. It is unavoidable for specific infectious diseases not to spread around the ward, and for this reason the affected ward is sometimes closed until the completion of the quarantine period.

Handwashing

As it is extremely easy to transmit germs from one patient to another it is of the utmost importance that the nurse washes her hands at numerous intervals while working with children.

Hands should be washed for one full minute, rinsed in antiseptic and dried thoroughly on an individual paper towel which is then disposed of.

The standards of cleanliness in the wards should be excellent, and each nurse must play her part in preventing the spread of infection.

Isolation of Infected Cases

There are certain infectious diseases which can be nursed in a cubicle or in the open ward. This necessitates 'barrier nursing' technique. Gastro-enteritis and infective hepatitis are two examples of such infectious disease.

The purpose of isolating the child is obviously to prevent the condition spreading to the other children and to the nurse herself.

If there is no cubicle available the child should be nursed in a corner of the ward near a window and a sink. A screen may be placed around the bed area to act as a reminder that the patient behind is infectious, but this does not keep the germs under control.

When nursing the child the nurse wears the gown provided. She should be particularly scrupulous about hand washing and hygiene. There should be a supply of gowns available for the nursing and medical staff.

The patient's requisites should be kept separately on a bed table within the bedside area, i.e. thermometer, dishes, cutlery, toys, fluid charts, toilet requisites etc. Wherever possible disposable equipment is used.

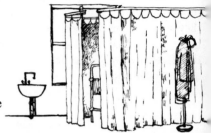

Two buckets are required to carry linen and napkins to the bathroom area for careful disposal. Adequate ventilation is required as this reduces the hazard of cross infection.

The patient stays in bed until treated satisfactorily for his condition. Lively attempts should be made to amuse him, as he will not have his young playmates, until he is free from infection.

Any local regulations about reporting the infectious disease should be adhered to as this information should be included in the nationwide statistical pattern.

49

Dismissal from Hospital

During the child's stay in hospital regular information will be given to the parents by the ward sister, or medical staff of the child's progress. When the time is approaching for the child to be dismissed from hospital, the parents should have reasonable warning. Most families are in close contact with their children in hospital. There is the odd family where the child in hospital has not been well visited, and in this case contact with the parents has to be made through the hospital medical social worker.

It is important that a member of the medical staff should interview the parents prior to discharge of the child in order that they obtain full understanding of their child's condition. A prescription may be given for drugs and an outpatient follow-up appointment made if required.

The mother of a young baby may be well advised to take him to her local child welfare clinic if a hospital appointment is not necessary.

The dietician may give advice on the diet.

The physiotherapist may advise on deep breathing exercises—or postural drainage so that the parents can cope efficiently at home.

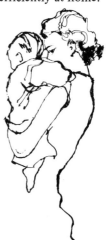

Although the child has usually been happy during his stay in hospital, it is with great joy, that the day approaches for him to leave with his parents.

IRREGULAR DISMISSALS

When parents wish to discharge their children from Hospital against medical advice, the nurse must deal with this situation calmly as the parents are invariably irate, and are feeling provoked.

It is expedient that a member of the medical staff, who will advise the parents, is notified. If they are still adamant about taking away their child, the consequences of irregular dismissal are explained and the child is allowed home.

An irregular dismissal form should be signed by the parents. This exonerates nursing and medical staff from any untoward consequences resulting from the parent's decision. A prescription may be given and a return date for an outpatient visit made if this is required

ACKNOWLEDGEMENTS

We would like to thank Professor Arneil for reading our proofs and Mr. Donaghy for pharmaceutical help.

A. M.
W. D.

PRIVATE AND CONFIDENTIAL

FLUID RECORD AND BALANCE CHART

Date.................................

Starting Time...............................Hours

Total at 12.00 hrs. or 24.00 hrs.........................

Surname ....

Other Names ....

Address ....

....

Hosp. No. ....

D. of B. ....

Sex ....

Clinic Ward ....

INTAKE in ml.

INITIALS		PARENTERAL				ORAL OR GASTROSTOMY	
	Time	Type	Level	Amount	Total	Type	Amount
TOTALS							

OUTPUT in ml.

URINE			DRAINAGE		OTHER		
Time	Urethra	Catheter	Right	Left	Vomit	Suction	Faeces

INSTRUCTIONS OR OBSERVATIONS

CRUDE BALANCE

POSITIVE/NEGATIVE

Index

abscess 40, 82
abdomen 39, 54
abdominal pain 43, 44, 52, 69
abdominal swelling 74
abducted position 24
accidents 128
Acetest 21
acetic acid 20
acetonuria 98
acid 21, 37
acquired heart disease 60, 62
A.C.T.H. 93
acyanotic 60
acyanotic congenital heart disease
    60, 62
adrenal gland 74
adrenaline 79
air 46
airway 76
albumin 52, 54
Albustix 20
alimentary disorders 34, 47
alimentary tract 29, 32, 33, 35
alkaline 21
allergy 79
'altered blood' 37
aluminium hydroxide gel 121
alveoli 75, 82
Ames test 20
anaemia 14, 38, 39, 44, 66, 102
anorexic 47, 81, 82, 94
antacid 37
antibiotics 41, 43, 44, 48, 52, 53, 69,
    77, 80, 81, 82, 83, 94
anti-convulsant drugs 90, 92, 93
antiseptic 23, 25
aorta 57
aortic valve 57, 61
aplastic anaemia 67
ascites 54
aseptic meningitis 94
aspirin 122

asthma 79
atrial septal defect 61
atrium 56, 57
axillae 45

'baby-sitter' 37
balance 87
barium-enema 29, 44
−meal 29
−swallow 29, 37
barrier nursing 44
bathing 111
B.C.G. 83
bed-rest 44, 63, 64, 69, 82, 84
bed-wetting 52
bile in urine 19
biliary atresia 103
bilirubin 100
biochemical 22
biopsy 74
bladder 51, 52
bladder puncture 52
blindness 85
blood 20, 43, 51, 52, 65
−'altered' 37
−calcium 26
−clotting 69
−culture 26
−disorders 31
−de-oxygenated 57
−examinations 23
−red cells 101
−in stools 44
−stream 34
−sugar 98
−vessels 50, 56
−white cells 85
bronchi 75, 76, 78
bronchioles 75
bronchitis 77, 78, 81
broncho-dilating 79
broncho-pneumonia 82

broncho-spasm 79
bones 49, 50
bone marrow 65, 71
bone marrow puncture 67, 72
bowel 36, 85, 125
—obstructions 37
—peristalsis 74
brain 87, 94
—tumour 72
breathlessness 40, 47, 58, 59, 63, 64
    77, 78, 79, 81, 82, 84
bruises 50, 68, 71

calcify 49
calcium 49
calories 12, 46, 99
capillaries 68, 75
carbohydrate 12, 38, 99, 102
carbon dioxide 53, 65, 75
cardiovascular system 56
'casts' 53
casualty 17
cells 65
—red blood 101
—white blood 85
cereal 14, 37
cerebellum 73, 87
cerebral palsy 96
cerebro-spinal fluid 27, 28, 94
cerebro-spinal space 28
chemicals 51
chicken pox 92
childhood 8, 9
chloride 65
chorea 62, 63
cleft-lip 47
—palate 47, 48
Clinistix 21
Clinitest 21
clot 65
coeliac disease 39, 47, 48, 67
colon 32, 44
coma 98
congenital heart disease 47, 58, 60,
    64, 62
conjunctivitis 83
constipated 36
contraction 36

convulsions 10, 18, 52, 76, 85, 88
    92, 94, 96, 99
cough 82
cretinism 90
croup 78
cryoprecipitate 70
C.S.F. 94
cyanosis 31, 57, 60, 62, 63, 64, 78,
    79, 81, 82, 92, 93

deformities 49
dehydration 43, 52, 78
diabetes 15
—insipidus 22
—mellitus 21, 98
diagnosis 16, 31
diaphragm 30
diarrhoea 18, 38, 39, 43, 44, 47
diet 15, 141
dentition 10
digestion 32, 33, 34, 38
digoxin 64, 121
discipline 106
diseases 31
dismissed 153
—irregular 154
'disturbed' child 22
diuresis 55, 64
drugs 31
—anti-convulsant 90, 92, 93
duodenum 32, 35
dwarfed 90
dying child 109
dysentery 43
dysuria 52

E.E.G. 93
elbow 23
electrolytes 26, 65
empyema 82
encephalitis 88
energy 12
enzymes 33, 34, 38, 39, 41
epistaxis 68
erythema-marginatum 62
—nodosum 83
erythrocytes 65
E.S.R. 26

'exchange transfusion' 101
external jugular vein 24, 25
eyes 54

face 54
facial paralysis 73
faeces 33
failure to thrive 45
falling 73
fat 12, 38
−in stools 38
father 12
fever 10, 52, 53, 76, 82
fibrocystic disease 41, 47
finger clubbing 58
feeding−bottle 12, 113
−breast 12
−difficulties 113, 117, 118, 119
−gavage 95
−graduated 43
gastric lavage 84
gavage feeding 95
gastro-enteritis 13, 31, 43, 47
gentian violet 42
globin 100
glucose 21, 98
gluten 39
glycosuria 98, 99
goitre 91
goitrous cretinism 91
grand mal seizures 92
groin 24, 36, 45
gut wall 34

hand-washing 43
haematuria 53, 69
haemoglobin 65, 66, 72, 100
haemolysis 67
haemolytic anaemia 67
haemophilia 69
haemorrhage 66, 68, 88
heads 112
headache 53, 73
hearing 87
heart 56
heart-disease 31, 58
−failure 60, 63, 64
−murmur 59, 60

−rate 10
−rhythm 63
height 9, 18
Henoch-Schonlein−Purpura 69
hepatomegaly 59
hiatus hernia 39, 31, 36, 47, 67
hibitane 23
history 16, 31
holes 60
hormones 65, 90
humidity 41, 76, 77, 78, 82
hydration 12, 34
hydrochloric acid 33
hygrometer 19
hypothermia 91
hypertrophied 35
hypoglycaemia 99

ileum 32
infant feeding 12
infancy 8
infantile spasms 93
infection 34, 42, 43, 44, 48, 52, 65
    72, 76, 123
−respiratory 47
−urinary 47
infectious diseases 151
infective hepatitis 102
ingestion of food 32
injection sites 123
intestinal obstruction 69
intestine 65
intra-cranial pressure 74
intravenous infusion 43, 44
intravenous fluids 146
insulin 21, 98
investigations 16, 31
iron 14, 65, 67
irradiation 29
irregular dismissal 154
isoprenaline 122
I.T.P. 68
I.V.P. 29, 30, 53
jaundice 31, 100
jejunal biopsy 39
jejunum 32, 39
joints 62, 69, 85

ketones 20, 21
kidney 20, 22, 51, 52, 54, 64, 74, 85
−disease 31

larynx 75, 78
legs 54
leucocytes 65
leukaemia 68, 71, 72
liver 34, 38, 66, 71, 74, 101, 102
liver disease 31
lumbar puncture 27, 28, 85, 94, 95
lumbar spine 28
lungs 57, 75
lymph nodes 65, 66, 71
lymphocytes 65

malabsorption syndrome 38, 40, 67
malignant disease 71
malignant tumour 74
Mantoux test 84, 85
marasmic 45
marrow 67
mastoid 80
meals 138
measles 92
measuring 130, 131
mechanised faults 35
medicine 31, 119, 120
medicine round 121
meningitis 27, 28, 31, 85, 94
−pyogenic 94
mental deficiency 47, 88, 93, 96
metabolism 90
methylated spirit 23
microscope 39, 52
micturating 51
milk 12
−full cream 12
−half cream 12
mitral valve 57
mixed feeding 14
molars 10
mongol 88
motor development 11
mouth 32, 75
M.S.S.U. 53
mucus 37, 40, 43, 44
mucous membranes 58

murmur 60, 62
muscles 87

nails 110
neonatal 8
nephritis 20, 53, 64
nephroblastoma 74
nephrotic syndrome 20, 54, 55
nervous system 87
neuro-surgeon 73
nose 75
−bleeds 68
−anaemia 66, 67
nutritional disorder 31

observation 7
obstruction 29, 35
oedema 31, 53, 54, 55, 59
oesophagus 32, 33, 37
oils 49
operation 31, 44, 48, 53, 61
ophthalmoscope 73
orthopaedics 31
otitis-media 80, 90
out patient 17
oxygen 57, 64, 75, 78, 81, 82, 148

pain 17
pale 39
pancreas 34, 38, 40, 41
Pancrex V capsule 121
Pancrex V powder 121
papilloedema 73
paralysis 73, 85
paroxysmal tachycardia 63, 64
penicillin 54, 69, 77
perinatal 8
petit mal seizure 93
pH of urine 21
pharynx 32, 33, 75
phenylketonuria 15, 90
physical examination 16
physiotherapy 41
plasma 65
platelet 65, 67, 68
pleural effusion 83
pleurisy 83

pneumonia 29, 40, 82
−broncho 82
poisoning 64
polydipsia 98
polyuria 98
potassium 64, 65
potty training 126
pre-natal brain damage 96
pre-school 8, 54
primary dentition 10
projectile vomiting 36, 37
protein 12, 14, 20, 38, 53, 54, 55, 65, 69
proteinuria 54, 55
psychological 44
psychomotor 9
puberty 9
pulmonary arteries 57
−valve 57
−veins 57
pulse 7, 59, 63, 125
puncture−bladder 52
−bone marrow 67, 72
purpura 67, 68, 71
pus 20, 52, 53, 82
−in urine 21
pyelonephritis 31, 52, 53
pyloric−muscle 36
−sphincter 35
−stenosis 31, 35, 36, 47, 48
−tumour 36
pylorus 36
pyogenic meningitis 94
pyrexia 81

radiography 83
radiologist 29
radio-opaque 29
radiotherapy 73, 74
rash 62, 69
red cells 26, 65, 100
rectal sedation 27
rectum 32, 44
regurgitation 37
remission 72
renal disease 20
renal failure 55
renal stones 21

renal tract 29
reporting 100
respiration 7, 12, 15, 125
respiratory disease 31, 46
respiratory infections 40, 41, 47
respiratory rate 10
respiratory system 75
rest 106
rhinitis 76
rheumatic fever 26, 64
rickets 29, 49, 50
ricketty rosary 49
rubella 88

sagittal sinus 24, 25
saline 43
saliva 33
salivary glands 32
salt 55
scurvy 15, 50
sedation 19, 27
sedative drugs 90
seizure 18
sensory nerves 87
septum 60
septicaemia 47
shigella 43
shock 43
sigmoidoscope 44
signs 16, 31
sinus arrhythmia 63
skin prick 23
skull 74
sleep 106
small bowel 32, 33, 34
smell 87
sodium 65
sodium chlorate 41
'spastics' 96
special drugs 121
specific gravity 19
spinal cord 87, 94
spleen 66, 71, 101, 102
squint 73
staggering 73
staphylococcus aureus 40
status asthmaticus 79
stenosed 61

stenosis—plumonary, aortic 61
steroid 55, 67, 72, 79, 122
stick tests 20
stilette 28
stomach 32, 33, 35, 36, 37
stomatitis 42
stools 18, 136
—blood in 44
—fat in 38
straight X-ray 29
straws—drinking 42
stridor 86
subcutaneous fat 45
sugar 20, 21
sulphonamides 122
sunlight 49
'suture lines' 73
swab 26, 53
sweat 12
sweat test 41
swelling 69, 91
sympathetic system 74
symptoms 16, 31
'systems' 31

tachycardia 59, 63, 64, 91
teat 42, 46
teeth 49, 111
telephone 108
temperature 7
test capsule 39
test feeding 36
throat 53, 62
thrush 42, 47
thyroid 65, 90
—gland 91
—hormone 91
tissues 12, 34, 50
toddler 8
tonsillitis 77
tonsils 77
tube feeding 82
tuberculosis 83
tumour 73, 74, 76
T.P.R 124
trachea 78
tracheostomy 78
transfusions 67

treatment 17
tricuspid valve 57
trypsin 41
twenty-four hour specimen 22
twitching 92, 93

ulcer 42, 66
ulcerative colitis 44
umbilical hernia 90
unconscious 27
under-feeding 45
—height 39
—weight 39
urea 26
ureter 51, 52
U.R.I. 76
urinalysis 19
urinary tract 51
—infection 20, 47, 92
urine 12, 51, 54
—containing bile 19
—containing blood 53, 69
—containing pus 21
—pH 21
—specimen 132

valves 57
—aortic 57, 61
—mitral 57
—pulmonary 57, 61
veins 57
venous blood 26
venepuncture 23
ventricle 56, 57
—left 57
ventricular septal defect 61
vertebrae 28
viral 78
virus 42, 76
visible peristalsis 36
vision 87
vitamins 14, 39, 41, 49, 50
vomiting 7, 10, 18, 31, 25, 36, 37,
    43, 45, 47, 52, 53, 64, 69, 73,
    85, 94, 98, 127
—projectile 36, 37

weaning 14

weight 9, 18, 55
weighing 130
wheezing 78, 79
white cells 65, 72
wind 115

wisdom teeth 10
wrist 29, 49

X-ray 29, 50, 61, 81, 84